CHRONICLES OF
A GYNAECOLOGIST

CHRONICLES OF A GYNAECOLOGIST

Tripti Sharan

BLOOMSBURY
NEW DELHI • LONDON • OXFORD • NEW YORK • SYDNEY

Bloomsbury Publishing India Pvt. Ltd
Second Floor, LSC Building No.4
DDA Complex, Pocket C – 6 & 7, Vasant Kunj
New Delhi 110070
www.bloomsbury.com

BLOOMSBURY and the Diana logo are trademarks of Bloomsbury Publishing Plc

First published in India 2016

ISBN 978 93 86141 42 2

Typeset by Manipal Digital Systems
Printed and bound in India by Replika Press Pvt Ltd

To find out more about our authors and books visit www.bloomsbury.com.
Here you will find extracts, author interviews, details of forthcoming
events and the option to sign up for our newsletters.

Dedicated to my father,
Mr P K Sharan
&
To the everlasting memory of my mother
Mrs Nirmala Sharan

*"Muted
they suffer
a frozen stupor.
An ignored presence,
yet awaiting a future .
Some random musings,
some scrambled letters.
Does it really make
me a writer better?"*

-Tripti Sharan

PREFACE

Chronicles of a Gynaecologist underlines the travails of a woman as she tries to hold on to her balance while passing through the various phases of life, coping with the demands of society, in addition to the ones her body places upon her. Pregnancy is not only an altered physiology, but also has profound psychological consequences. Occasionally, these changing body dynamics are far reaching. The author tries to decipher the conundrum of a woman's life as she pauses at each step.

The book is also a reflection of the author's journey as a doctor. The stories have been inspired by real life incidents. The author has indulged her imagination to turn it into a soul stirring fiction.It explores issues ranging from something as important and largely preventable as medical complications of pregnancies, to touching upon the rampant superstitions and myths surrounding them, to the influence of quacks and preachers on a woman's psyche. It also deals with postpartum depression, things still regarded as taboo such as altered sexual orientation and intersex, as well as delves into shocking and serious eventualities such as rape, incest and perversions that threaten to tear apart the spirit of any woman. We live in the era of changing morality and social values. Every story raises a curtain and promises to be a revelation.

Some deeply entrenched beliefs, some dogmatic attitudes – the stories largely speak of the trauma and struggles of women from various walks of life, the concomitant defences commonly resorted to, and not infrequently, the mounting retaliatory offences.

Women across the globe continue to suffer from pregnancy related complications. India has an astoundingly high maternal mortality rate – a staggering 174 per 100,000 live births (2015).

As Mahmoud Fathalla, past president of the International Federation of Gynecology and Obstetrics (FIGO) said:

'Women are not dying because of diseases we cannot treat. They are dying because societies have yet to make the decision that their lives are worth saving.'

It's the time to take the wake up call. A smiling woman is the face of a vibrant society. A vibrant society is a proof that civilization is still alive. Let's shed off age-old beliefs and bias, some taboos and some trials, and spread a smile on her face.

ACKNOWLEDGEMENTS

This is most definitely not my story.

A story 'sits' in front of me and pours out her heart. How can one, who beholds a pen, not write about her? Yet I am just a medium in 'His' chosen plans.and I thank the Almighty for giving me the opportunity to share 'her' tales with the world.

I thank my parents for blessing me with the 'sense and the sensibilities'. Their selflessness sowed the seeds of empathy in my heart. Their gentleness and kindness has acted as the torch whose light I want to spread into the world.

It all started in the crowded Khan Market where I sat with the co-authors of my previous book on poems *The Dewdrops... a journey begins*. What brew that day was not merely coffee beans, and the idea of writing stories took birth in that buzzing café. I was most vehemently in denial, yet here I am acknowledging them for their thoughtful advice – thanks Abhijit and Neeti for the push in the right direction.

When a doctor writes, what comes out is sometimes more of a prescription. I acknowledge the untiring efforts of noted author and psychiatrist, Dr Ashok Prasad, and friend and bestselling author, Alcatraz Dey, in mulling over my amateurish writings. I demanded their opinion at the most inappropriate and inconvenient moments, totally disregarding the civilities of a 'proper' time. It's their patience that turned my erratic and sometimes disjointed thoughts into a powerful narration.

My alma mater, my medical school Gajra Raja Medical College, Gwalior, where it all began, the hospitals where I have worked till now, my friends and colleagues who have been my partners in this amazing journey, bear the testimony to all that I write. They are the background to all my stories. I am just a moderator. They have taught me more than my medical textbooks. They are my life and I owe them so much more.

My stories lay struggling in a folder under the weight of 'The Documents' on my computer, till I met Deepesh Bhardwaj. He is the reason my book could jiggle out and breathe free. I could never get around to thanking him, simply because words were never enough. But then words are all that I have!

Praveen and Nitin have been nothing short of miracles to me. Bloomsbury happened because they came at the right time. I thank my publishers, Bloomsbury India, for believing in my stories and sharing my zeal. Their enthusiasm and faith kept me going even when I would nurse doubts and get jittery. Debangana, my dear editor! There have been times when I have really sympathised with her. She was the one at the receiving end of my intellectual 'avatar'. My pen has a tendency to take 'U' turns, flip over and leave a trail of cuts and bruises. I owe her more than a free check-up. (Though I hope she never needs that!) But seriously, they have delivered my baby.

My batchmate, and later my husband too, Dhiren Gupta, I know will not read any of my stories. Yet he understands the gist of the stories and lets me write undisturbed. For that I can never thank him enough. I hope he has forgotten all about the mysterious and frequent disappearance of the television remote.

My children, Aryan and Manav, suffered my absence, and it's their time that was forsaken for writing, yet the beautiful children never complained. (I am forgetting the little treats I had to bribe them with!) I adore them for the unconditional love and casual hugs they throw my way

My sister, Dr Rachna Varma, has been unequivocal in her zeal to promote me and my books, to the extent that her friends are now wary of a sister who keeps coming up with a book. She has worked hard behind the screen. I can never thank her enough for her unwavering support. May she keep being showered by my books.

I am blessed to have friends like Dipanker Mukherjee, Yaseen Anwar, and Sumit G Sehgal, who have always been ready to help 'a doctor' understand the workings of the writing industry. They have always been just a phone call away, forever ready to lend an ear to a rueful writer. I acknowledge their generosity.

My father-in-law, Dr J B Gupta, endured my drafts without complaining. He always believed that I would be a writer one day. This book is a daring proof of his conviction. I can never thank him enough.

My extended family and friends are the ones who bore the onslaught of my writings. I thank them all, even for the undeserving 'likes' they put on social media. Their constant motivation has been the driving force behind this book.

And what would be the world of a writer if not for those precious RAMs and bytes. Microsoft Word made up for my lack of formal English classes. It is the world's best English teacher, always ready to correct my spellings and punctuations, and restructure my sentences. It never reprimanded, just quietly underlined; blue, green, and sometimes red! The world of software has made it possible to write, edit, store and send documents across the same day, without getting stuck in any messy traffic. I thank the technology that has made life so much simpler for the writer.

And how do I thank the main protagonists of my stories! They have sat silently on a stool in my chamber, lay in distress in the wards, sometimes speaking brazenly, sometimes staying hidden in the shadows. I bow to the 'essence of a woman', a power that has carried us through civilisations. They have given me the lesson of life! I have come across so many of them; saw a woman inside me, too, yet I am always left amazed at their resilience that has withstood so much bias and so many trials. I can't name them, but I acknowledge the contribution of each one of them in my enlightenment.

I shall always be indebted to the souls of those who left so early in the journey of life and could not be part of this moment. I deeply regret that we, as a civilized society, could not save their precious lives. They suffered in the hands of an apathetic system, yet their story shall go a long way in making us aware and sensitive to their unfortunate saga.

In the end, I thank you, my reader, for giving me your precious time. You have made it possible for me to share my experiences. I hope you find them interesting and thought provoking.

'May we understand her better, and may she achieve her rightful place one day!'

Amen!

Tripti Sharan
triptisharan2003@yahoo.co.in
http://www.facebook.com/writer.tripti

CONTENTS

1
THE RAPE VICTIM - MY TRYST WITH JUSTICE

"Eyes that forgot to see,
Eyes that forgot to weep;
They never smiled,
They never lived,
Yet they follow me…"

The streets of the city wore a deserted look. Heat was the new Taliban forcing women to wear a *hijab*. It was a common sight to see girls riding a two-wheeler, draping their *chunni* in such a way that only their eyes were visible. The wiser ones preferred to stay indoors, but the lesser fortunate ones, like a doctor on duty, didn't have much choice. Braving the heat, I entered the premises of the hospital, and was immediately welcomed by a gush of cool air. Almost all the buildings in the city carried the legacy of the royal family of Gwalior. The Kamla Raja Hospital, meant for only women and children, was literally our residence, as true to its meaning, our residency days hardly left time for anywhere else. However, now in the final year of post-graduation, we had become quite accustomed to our weird lives.

As I entered the casualty ward, I saw a policeman waiting inside. He looked relieved to see me. We were quite familiar with these policemen and, at times, I felt that their job was as tough as ours, if not tougher. Like us, they had difficult working conditions and graveyard shifts. Add to it, they were always in the public eye; the public that was forever in desperate situations and quick to judge.

They often brought those involved in police cases to the hospital for medical check-ups. We were wary of them. Not that we didn't sympathise, but doing such cases (we called them medicolegal cases) meant leaving our routine work. Add to it, loads of clerical work and getting caught in legal procedures or logjam. So we ended up giving these policemen our most unwelcome smile. Well, that never stopped them! I noticed that the policeman was holding out a paper in his hand. With slight trepidation I took it from him. It was a summon from the court for a rape case in which the victim was brought to us for medical check-up a year back. Her name did not ring any bell. How was one supposed to remember a case done so long back? Unfortunately, that's the pace at which the judiciary moves in our country.

Many of my seniors had told me about their courtroom experiences. The doctor was a neutral witness. The courts were generally courteous and helpful. Sometimes it did get dangerous when influential people were involved, but generally it went off smoothly. This was my first summon and I could feel a tinge of excitement creeping in. The court hearing was a week later, so I had time to check the case from the records. As I browsed through the papers, a woman with frozen eyes entered my mind. I could vividly recall the fear lurking in her eyes – how they stared but saw nothing. It took me back all those months to that fateful day…

There was a persistent knock at the door and I could see a policewoman peering through the partially closed door, 'Ma'am! Please see this woman. She is in a lot of distress.'

We had a love-hate relationship with the police.

'Sudha Rani, you always say that. Just because you want to get free quickly, it doesn't mean that I leave everything and come rushing at your command.' I was a little wary and made no bones about it. She still persisted. It was unlike her, as she usually left the 'cases' she brought in the casualty, and went on to do her errands. I was neither keen nor easily impressed as I had lately seen many fabricated cases, and they wasted a lot of our time.

However, as I glanced, I saw a small, thin, and dark woman, wearing a torn saree and some ugly bruises on her face, quietly perched in the corner. I called her but she didn't respond. The policewoman gave her a gentle shove and she walked inside towards me.

As she drew nearer, I could easily see the stains of dried tears on her cheeks. She was walking with difficulty.

I asked her, 'Do you know that this examination can go against you? Would you still want to go ahead with it?'

She kept quiet. I was in a hurry and was getting a little irritated, too. I had to take her consent before proceeding.

Sudha Rani came to my rescue, '*Haan bol de, beta.*' ('Say yes, child.')

She simply stared at me blankly. I took out the papers and, prompted by the policewoman, she wordlessly gave her thumb impression.

Sudha Rani said, 'Madamji, *unmarried larki hai* (she is an unmarried girl). She's been raped by two men!'

I winced. After bearing the trauma of rape, she now had to go through the medical check-ups.

Something about her whole demeanour was making me uncomfortable and, against my better judgement of not ever being personal, I asked her, 'What happened?'

She raised her eyes once again but said nothing.

Sudha Rani interrupted, 'Madam, *ye kuch nahi bolegi. Aap complaint padh lo.*' ('Madam, she will not say anything. You read the complaint filed by her.')

I took out the report and quickly went through it. This 22-year-old woman was on her way back home when she was attacked by two men. They were from the neighbouring village. She was raped by them and later dumped near a road. A passer-by noticed her and took her to a police station. It was indeed horrifying. However, more than the crime, it was the language of the complaint filed by her that disgusted me. It was written in crude Hindi and sounded almost vulgar. I accepted that a majority of our population could still not understand English, but just going through the statement made my hair stand on end. I shivered as I tried to imagine a woman writing it, especially before the notorious policemen. How demeaning to have it read in front of her family! Was there no other way to make it less humiliating?

'Why do you people make them write in such a vulgar language?' I vented it out all on poor Sudha Rani.

She shrugged, '*Kya karen? Aur kaise likhenge? Zurm bhi to bahut vulgar hai na.*' ('What to do? How else to write? The crime is also extremely vulgar.')

The two accused had also been sent for a medical examination. It didn't make me feel any better.

Her torn clothes and the signs of injury on her body were testimony to her plight. Painful blisters and bruises had already started forming. It was difficult to make her lie down. The fear in her eyes spoke volumes, and only after a lot of coaxing could she lie down for an examination. There were a lot of injury marks on her private parts, too. Probing further, I was surprised to notice that she was still a virgin! Medically, an intact hymen did not rule out sexual interference, nor a torn hymen proved previous sexual intercourse. Not deliberating much, I simply noted it down and completed the rest of the examination. Her clothes were sealed and sent for forensic examination along with the vaginal swabs and slides. Once finished, she was free to go. A tired-looking, dhoti-clad man waited outside, probably her father. He folded his hands in gratitude and soon they were out of the hospital…

A cry from the adjoining labour room jolted me back to the present. Maybe she had let go of her fears and learned to smile again.

The week passed quickly and soon came the day for the first attendance in the court. I was getting a little apprehensive but I pushed away my nagging doubts. I didn't want to dampen my enthusiasm.

The district court was buzzing with activity. Everywhere, there were harassed-looking people scuttling behind their lawyers, carrying a trail of overloaded files, or should I say 'justice', in their hands. I was used to seeing handcuffed patients in the hospital too, but they still made me curious. Many could easily pass off as one of our poor workers; not quite like the villains we see in the movies. I often wondered if indeed there was a Prem Chopra scheming inside them, or were they like the angry young man Amitabh Bachchan, wrongly accused and suffering silently? Maybe this came from watching too many movies!

My uncle had accompanied me, and he directed me to the courtroom. The large hall was precariously bare. Broken benches and shabby interiors graced a hall that had probably seen better days. A large, ancient-looking fan making rude noises attracted my attention. I smiled… I had seen one such fan in my grandfather's house. The imposing fan, despite its size and loud noise, appeared to be under a lot of strain and moved slowly. Just like the judiciary of our country! The dirty walls, the tattered doors and windows, and the subdued yellow lights were probably a testimony to so many courtroom dramas. The images of the impressive courtrooms that had lingered so long in my mind, bid a silent adieu. Definitely not an *Insaf ka Tarazu* (Scales of Justice) kind of filmy scene. The only similarity was the lady with her eyes covered, holding the *tarazu* (scales) in her hand. Unfazed and unperturbed she stood there, for she didn't really see anything.

There were a few people sitting on the benches, waiting for their turn. All of us had been given serial numbers. Mine was the first, and I had been given a file containing the medical report of the victim. Now, only the judge needed to arrive.

I looked around, hoping to see the woman, and saw a vaguely familiar dhoti-clad man standing next to a lawyer. He saw me looking at him and gave me a hesitant smile. I made my way towards them. He folded his hands and looked at me gently.

The lawyer bowed slightly and said, 'I am her lawyer. He is my client's father.'

'How is she?' I could hardly stop myself.

'She's no more.'

The father looked at me with moist eyes. I was shocked, gripped by an acute sense of loss.

'She had grown very depressed in the weeks that followed and had lost interest in everything. She was not eating much, either. The repeated visits to the police station and the court took its toll. One day, she fell ill with high grade fever. We thought it was a normal fever, but it turned out to be brain fever. Despite our best efforts, she could not be saved. Now my only wish is to punish those responsible for her death.' His small frame shook with silent grief.

The lawyer was very quiet. With the victim no more, had he lost steam?

Suddenly, there was a flurry of activity and another lawyer, surrounded by a group of people, entered the courtroom. He appeared restless and was moving his hands frantically as he spoke. There were two men wearing dirty clothes trailing him. I presumed them to be the accused. The lawyer was patting and reassuring them. He looked around before sitting down on a bench a few rows ahead of me. The group appeared to be engrossed in a heated discussion interrupted by occasional grunts from the lawyer. Suddenly, he got up looking at his watch and noticed me sitting a few yards away. He glanced at me insolently. I shifted uncomfortably in my seat.

'The *doctorni*?' He laughed sarcastically and patted the man next to him, speaking a bit too loudly, probably for my benefit.

I disliked him immediately. His whole attitude exuded arrogance. One expects to see the best behaviour and discipline in the room of Your Honour!

I was spared further glances as the judge arrived, and soon the room fell into some kind of order. The judge took his place. Someone sat beside the judge, in front of the typewriter. On being called, I moved into the area which I believe was the witness box. It was in the centre, just in front of the judge. Immediately, I was surrounded by people. Even the accused stood there, peering at me. The judge, being at a higher level, could still watch me. This was not how my first court appearance should have been, but I still tried to maintain my composure. I touched the holy book *Gita*, as if drawing some strength from it.

'You can start.' The judge asked me to read out my report. Feeling a bit confident, I started. Immediately, I was interrupted by the defence lawyer, 'Madamji, in Hindi!'

I fumbled, but realized that it was a norm and started again, this time in Hindi. As I spoke, a typewriter recorded every word I uttered. I managed to get through the complains and the gynaecological history. I chose to ignore the occasional scoffing sounds. However, my mask of bravery threatened to slip when it came to reading the examination part.

The line 'secondary sexual characters and her pubic and axillary hair well developed' swam in front of me. How do I describe her anatomy, her sexuality, in Hindi? I felt like kicking myself for writing such details. My self-reproach didn't make me feel any better, and I looked at the judge, silently appealing. He nodded, much to the displeasure of the defence lawyer. Relieved, I went on using medical terms in English to describe the injury marks on her body and genital areas. As I moved further to her internal check-up, I mentioned her virginal status to the court a little hesitatingly. I silently cursed myself for being so brutally honest.

The defence lawyer jumped at that. 'Hold it, madam. You said the hymen is intact?' I nodded.

'But she has been raped by two men!' He flung his arms all around, as if expecting approval from everyone. 'How can it be so, if she has been raped?' he asked sarcastically. He persisted in using chaste Hindi, maybe just to intimidate me.

I was now nervous. Pitted against a lawyer who wanted to win at any cost, I wished I could look squarely at his face and ask him to go to hell.

However, pulling myself together, I managed to say, 'According to the definition, it is not something necessary to constitute rape.'

He jumped at that. 'Madam, leave aside definitions. This is not a classroom. *Seedhi, sachi bhasha mein batao. Agar rape hoga, toh hymen rupture hoga ki nahi?*' ('Tell me in a simple language. If there has been a rape, will the hymen rupture or not?')

I was getting flustered, but still managed to insist, 'The mere touching of inner parts by the male organ can constitute rape.'

He was getting agitated, 'OK, *yeh batao mujhe – agar koi do aadmi zabardasti apna male organ kisi female organ ke andar dale*, will the hymen remain intact? (OK, tell me this – if two men forcibly insert their male organ into a female organ, will the hymen remain intact?) Yes or no?'

Horrified by his audacity, and the crude Hindi he used, I staggered. A sea of unsympathetic faces loomed around me. I looked at the judge and the other lawyer in silent appeal.

'Legally...'

My voice trailed off as he interrupted my last effort almost ferociously, 'Madam, *legal-wegal aap hum pe choro.*' ('Madam, leave the legalities to us.') He repeated the whole offensive statement once again in Hindi, emphasizing every word with sadistic pleasure. 'Yes or no?'

I fumbled. My courage was slowly deserting me. This was turning into a nightmare.

He again shouted, 'Yes or no?'

I literally jumped and said, 'Yes.'

Even before I had finished, the typist had marked 'yes' on the papers. Something inside me broke. I started again, 'But, sir ...'

The lawyer had already turned towards the judge. Wearing a broad smile, he said, 'I don't need to ask anything else, Your Honour. Your turn...' He turned towards the victim's lawyer.

The lawyer, who seemed to have already accepted his defeat, said, 'I don't want to ask her anything, Your Honour.'

The judge thanked me and asked me to leave. The crowd burst into applause. Nobody could see a young female doctor reeling in shock there. I couldn't get past my sense of failure; so powerful that it was killing me. I still marvel at how I didn't break into tears.

Moving past the crowd, I saw the victim's father standing in a corner, his hands still folded. Eyes brimming with anguish, I looked at him. He was the only person who understood the plea in my unshed tears. Now I could live the fear, the loss of life, in those haunting eyes. If those few minutes spent there were so traumatic, how had she survived the whole ordeal? No wonder she was broken. However, with it, the realization hit home that, today, she had lost because of me. How could I ever respect myself? If only I had not succumbed so easily! My regret was soon getting replaced by an intense anger. Is this how justice was delivered in this country? Wasn't being raped once, not enough? Was rape of the soul not as important as that of the body? How could those, who delivered justice, be so unjust?

I turned back. I had to see the judge once again. Suddenly, I felt my arms being seized. My uncle, who was sitting in one of the back rows and, thankfully, had not heard much of the trial, held me back.

'Please! I want to talk to the judge. I have to explain to him.'

He laughed at my naivety.

'The judge is already on his next case. It is neither proper, nor does it make much sense, talking to him now. Forget the case!' he gently advised me.

I was still fuming, but as I walked outside the premises, I accepted the futility of my action. The judgement had been delivered, even though justice had been denied. Truth had been proven wrong; a lie had survived and won. I had to live with that on my conscience. My trauma in the court didn't have any name. Yet, my weak disposition would haunt me forever. Maybe one day, I would be able to face the accusation in her eyes. Maybe, one day I would plead guilty in front of a pair of eyes which had stopped living but followed me forever...

2
THE SILENT RETREAT

"Nobody heard, nobody cared,
For the silent retreat
of that solitary beat!
Nobody knew when it quietly
ceased to be…"
(From my poem *The Silent Retreat,* published in the book *The Dewdrops… a journey begins*)

The labour room is easily the most dynamic place in a hospital. It is the only place in the complex where the serenity of the hospital is broken by the 'first cry', leading to much rejoice and celebration. Relatives pace the floor, anxiously awaiting the arrival of a new life, at times even blocking the entry to the labour room. There were strict instructions to not allow them to hover around the main door, but rather to make them wait patiently in the waiting area. However, I discovered that Indians are not easily put in a line, when I was about to enter and noticed a crowd gathered just outside the labour ward. With mild trepidation, I pushed open the door. I was surprised to see policemen inside, and a distraught Dr Payal trying to explain something, frantically. I reached her side quickly.

'What happened?' I looked at her questioningly, but she signalcd mc to wait.

Not wanting to disturb, I decided to wait for her in the duty room. Soon, a hassled Dr Payal walked inside.

'Phew! What a duty!'

She just flopped on the bed and went on to narrate the unfortunate events which had unfolded in the darkness of the night.

'I was looking forward to finishing off my rounds and going back home. There had been about thirty deliveries in the eighteen-hour-long night shift, and my tired nerves were now screaming in protest. However, before winding up, I had to shift all the delivered patients to the post-natal ward. As I reached the last bed in the corner, it was unusually quiet, unlike other beds. The patient was reclining on the bed, holding her baby.'

'Can you keep the baby on the bed and lie down, I said. She was reluctant, but complied.'

'The baby looked very pale and there was something disturbing about it. As I touched it, I was shocked to find it lifeless. I raised an alarm and soon other doctors and staff rushed in. The baby was declared dead after all efforts to resuscitate it failed. A healthy newborn died inside the labour room in her mother's arms, without any antecedent cause and precipitating factor!'

'How did this happen, I shouted at the patient.'

'The patient feigned ignorance about anything. "Pata nahi, madamji. Humne to dhoodh pila ke sula diya tha." ("I don't know, madam. I fed her milk and put her to sleep.") She kept on insisting that the baby was sleeping.'

'Her mother-in-law was also there till an hour back. She was called in. "*Hey Bhagwaan! Ye kaise ho gaya? Lakshmi mata humse ruth gayi.*" ("Oh God! How did this happen? Goddess Laxmi has walked away from our house.") She broke into a long wail, thumping her chest and screaming hysterically.'

'Soon, a crowd started gathering. "The standard of government hospitals has gone down. Imagine all this happening inside the labour room." They grumbled about the poor quality of care given by doctors, and negligence in the hospitals. That bugged my tired senses.'

'The baby had been handed over to the mother about five hours back in perfectly healthy condition. If she or her attendants couldn't find anything amiss, and still the baby died, it was their negligence, not that of the doctors. This was her third baby. She was not even an inexperienced mother, I answered back tersely.'

'It was disgusting to see shock replace sympathy on the faces of many onlookers. Somehow, her being a baby girl made things more acceptable. It was strange that the family was not overtaken by grief. Their cold acceptance of this unexpected loss was, indeed, suspicious.'

Dr Payal finished her story. The signs of distress were clearly visible on her face.

This was an unexplained death, so the police was informed. They arrived and started their investigation. They questioned the family, and the doctors and staff on duty. Everyone was eyed with suspicion. Sudden cot-deaths were known because of accidental smothering by the mother, and also sometimes by milk aspiration, but the police didn't want to rule out foul play. The baby had a red mark slowly forming over the neck, suggestive of a ligature mark, which raised the possibility of strangulation. The body was sent for post-mortem. In the meantime, the police decided to investigate the scene of crime further. They clicked pictures and spoke to eye witnesses.

One of the policemen entered the delivery room. It was an invasion of our private area, but we didn't have any choice.

'How do you deliver babies?' The policeman looked around insolently.

A little disconcerted, we briefly described the procedure.

He quipped, 'So, maybe the doctor could also strangulate the baby while delivering?'

His flippancy was enough to send our blood gushing in anger, but we decided to ignore him. We had had enough dramas for the day so we let that pass. Thankfully, he did not trouble us any more with his stupid queries.

The case kept on firing the imagination of people and was a hot topic of debate at most corners. There were some who were almost too vocal of the misfortunes of having a third female child. Stories of female infanticide, rampant in some parts of Rajasthan and Haryana, kept resurfacing. A baby is a sign that our civilization is still alive. Could the gender of a new born baby justify its death at the hands of its own parent?

The labour room was flooded with visitors and, with difficulty, we doused the curiosity of everyone. We were already getting late for our rounds and outdoor clinics.

There was a big chaos outside the clinic. No sooner had we started that a thin woman was pushed inside by her angry husband, amidst sounds of protest.

'You wait outside. Please come by turns only,' the OPD nurse shouted at him.

'My wife is not well and we cannot keep waiting forever,' he replied angrily as he pushed his way inside. She actually looked frail, so I asked her to lie down.

'She is twenty-three years old, and into her ninth month of pregnancy. We got her check-up done once in the village dispensary, but they referred her here,' her husband grumbled.

She was indeed pale and her recent haemoglobin was just three grams. That was barely enough to keep her alive and she was pregnant on top of that. Such a low haemoglobin meant years of poor nutrition and neglect. Even the livestock in the villages were better looked after. They didn't look very poor either. Her husband appeared healthy enough.

'Why can't you take care of yourself?' we reprimanded her.

'Madam, I hardly get any time. There is so much work at home. We have a big family,' she said slowly. Her domestic chores were more important than her health.

'Why didn't you see a doctor earlier?'

'Doctor *sahib*, our women deliver at home by our village *dai* (midwife). It's not our custom to take womenfolk to hospitals. I at least took her to the dispensary yesterday.' The husband was quite proud of the fact that he had brought her to a hospital when the majority of women delivered at home in his village.

'Our *dai* has been delivering our women for the last two generations. She never told me of any such danger and had rather warned me that the city doctors scared people unnecessarily and complicated things.'

'Obviously, if cattle and goats could deliver in the fields easily, why not women?'

The sarcasm was, however, lost on the insensitive man. He kept on grumbling for having to wait so long. He could wait nine months for a proper visit to a hospital, but couldn't wait for a few minutes in the hospital.

'Look, she needs urgent admission and blood transfusion.'

'*Kyun?*' ('Why?') The husband didn't understand the need for either. It was a struggle explaining the gravity of the situation to him.

'She will die if you do not.' When we persisted, he agreed.

'*Thik hai* madamji, *aap mangwa do. Hum mol pe lenge.*' ('OK madam, you order the blood. We will buy it.')

'The hospital doesn't accept blood bought from outside. It is nothing more than a *Ruhafza*, a soft drink, with the possibility of infections. You will have to donate, or ask somebody to donate.'

'*Main khoon dene laga, toh kaam kaun karega?*' ('If I start donating blood, then who will work?') He was already regretting coming here. He just would not hear of it.

'OK, then you will have to sign the negative consent and take responsibility if anything goes wrong.'

After a lot of arguments with other doctors, and nurses also scolding him, he agreed for blood transfusion but at a condition!

'I will inform her brothers. Let them come and donate blood for her, and then I will admit her,' he declared generously.

We were taken aback. She was married to him for five years – the dutiful, undemanding wife who would bear him kids. Didn't she merit even a drop of life from her husband? All the while the woman kept quiet, her face hidden in her saree. We marvelled at her tolerance. How easily they succumb to the norms dictated by their husbands!

He sensed our scowl and explained, 'Actually the first delivery is the responsibility of her father. We follow these customs in our village.' Of course, there was no custom of humanity followed in his village. It was pointless arguing with him. He didn't realize that it was indeed a miracle that his wife was still alive. They were sitting on the top of a volcano. Anytime the system would decompensate and she would collapse.

'You at least get her admitted. The hospital would arrange blood and, in the meantime, you can arrange the donors.' We insisted on admission, assuring him, but he refused to budge.

She was to be admitted only when her family came in. We had no choice but to take a negative consent for admission. They signed the papers willingly and walked out of the hospital, the obedient wife silently towing behind her selfish husband. We doubted he would come back and looked sadly at her retreating back.

We were living in the capital city. If such things happened here, the condition in other parts of the country was unimaginable. Were we indeed a sadistic nation with no right to call ourselves a civilized society?

For ages, women had suffered discrimination. From Sita to Draupadi, in every saga, women were made the epitome of sacrifice, all in the name of *dharma*. Strangely, in a country where motherhood was always celebrated, womanhood was not even a concern.

The next few days saw the police visiting and interrogating people. Finally, the patient whose newborn baby girl had died was arrested on charges of murder. The mother-in-law was also arrested on the same charges. They did their dirty work in our hospital, so we all became either witnesses or suspects. This meant endless courtroom dramas for us. In all the din and flurry of events, we had forgotten the severely anaemic patient.

A week later, I was on emergency duty.

'A patient with severe anaemia had come in labour. Her heart could not cope with the stress of delivery and failed. She collapsed and is very critical. Chances of her survival are very dim.' My grim faced colleague told me as she handed over the patients. I had a bad intuition about this patient and went to see her in the ICU. She was battling for her dear life. Multiple units of blood had been pumped in, but how could you reverse the chronic strain to the heart and tissues that had been deprived of oxygen for so long. The baby had miraculously survived. As I was leaving, I saw a familiar looking man standing outside the ICU. Yes, he was the same person who had taken his wife forcibly away from the hospital that day.

'So you admitted your wife well in time,' I told him sarcastically.

'What to do, madamji? Her brothers took so much time in coming.' Nonplussed, he went on complaining about her brothers.

The silent wife, whose husband refused to accept his responsibility, succumbed to her fate a few hours later. Her death left an overriding feeling of guilt and helplessness. If only we had somehow not let her go that day. However, we could not hold a patient against her will. Unfortunately, here the will of the husband surpassed any will of her own. Another victim added to anaemia, a leading cause of maternal death in our country. One just needs good diet and proper medical care to tackle it, but it kills remorselessly because the country is helpless against the deep-running ignorance and traditions.

As I came outside the ICU to finish the formalities, I couldn't hold back my jibe to the husband, 'People like you should be arrested. You have not lost anything! Now that she is no more, you will marry again. Along with a new wife, you get a new motorcycle and a fat dowry.'

He replied innocently, '*Naah* madam, it is not so simple any more… very difficult to marry in villages these days.'

I felt like hitting some sense into him. The woman deserved at least some tears for her selfless service to him, but here he was, already thinking about his remarriage. There was no trace of any guilt or remorse on his face. The immediate cause of death might have been anaemia, but the antecedent cause of death was lack of care, and neglect. If indeed we could sue such families and hold them accountable for gross negligence. A group of relatives were sitting in a separate corner, wiping away their tears. They were probably her parents and brothers. Maybe in their village, the custom was only for the parents and siblings to grieve; the husband's family was not to be bothered

A woman died of a preventable cause. A newborn was strangulated by her mother because of her gender. Probably, she too would have met a similar fate later on. Both were victims of the same patriarchal mindset that refuses to treat women as equals. Their deaths laid bare the hypocrisy that throbs in our country when it comes to treating our womenfolk. We have no qualms in accepting technology when we wear modern clothes, use modern methods of communication, and use hi-tech gadgets for our comfort, but when it comes to a woman's health, we become all-traditional. A strange country we live in!

And we had failed. As a civil society, we were responsible for their deaths. As a country, we stood shamed, once again.

3
SHADES OF GREY - PART I

"But sometimes when the dusk draws,
And the shadows fall,
Veils are lifted on all the flaws.
Gone is the time for pretense,
Creeps silently, a sinister silence…"
(Adapted from my poem *Hey! Am I really bad?* published in the
book *The Dewdrops… a journey begins*)

The worst part about being a gynaecologist is to be a standby
for the non-existing sex therapist. Few people appreciate the
difference. Living in the land of *Kamasutra* that still frowns
upon sex, the hypocrisy of the society teaches people to hide
and do things undercover. And underneath this, breathes
the unmet needs of the people. Suppressed desires have dire
consequences, reflected in the rising graph of sexual crimes
and violence. People across all ages throng to the internet to
make themselves sexually-literate. A sound professional advice
remains the rarest of all resources. And a gynaecologist is the

best choice in most situations. In a changing society, with the temptation from a readily available virtual world, morality has become merely a lack of opportunity. Secret liaisons, unfulfilled desires, the need to curb down even normal needs, sometimes lead to hospitals in grave situations.

It was not that I was getting philosophical for no reason. Something had pissed me off completely. A gentleman was pestering me with his crude curiosities, bordering on vulgarity. The first time he called me, I was in the middle of a party. He gave my colleague's reference, a much senior and respectful consultant, before asking abruptly, 'Is it all right to use an expiry date condom?'

'An expiry date condom!' I repeated, much to the shocked expressions of those surrounding me.

I hurriedly excused myself from the group before asking him what exactly he meant. If he was so concerned, he should have checked that before, for God's sake! And if it still bothered him, the least he could do now was buy an emergency contraceptive pill. Of course, he should check the expiry date of that too, or else he could simply wait for the consequences till the next month. Normally I didn't get goaded easily, but I definitely didn't like being embarrassed in front of my friends. If only people respected the privacy of doctors, too. In the West, one can't dream of calling a doctor at just any time. We love comparing ourselves with them, but in such situations, we conveniently go the typical Indian way.

If I thought my flippancy had seen the end of him, I was in for a surprise. He had made me, invariably, a lending shoulder to his careless behaviour. Few days later, I got a call from him again. This time, it was only two minutes before midnight. A different time and a slightly different complain. The woman in question was in severe pain. He had bitten her off. He wasn't in the least apologetic, but wanted to know why this happened and if this could be serious. How was one supposed to answer this and assess it over a telephone? I refused to talk to him and asked for the woman. She actually sounded distressed, so I asked her to take a painkiller and rush to the hospital. As expected, they never turned up.

I brought this to the notice of my senior colleague next day, who apologized and agreed that this guy was a little weird. He had recently divorced, and was now in a relationship with a much younger girl. That was none of my business and it didn't explain his behaviour at all. I didn't mind seeing a woman in my clinic even with vague complains, but I would be damned if I had to listen to such complains over the telephone, that too at a completely indecent time. My colleague promised to convey my displeasure, and make sure he visited me in the hospital, if at all needed.

True to what he had promised, this gentleman walked into my clinic few days later. And beside him walked the girl. He met me with the familiarity of friends meeting after a long time. I had promised myself I wouldn't get irritated with him, and that really helped. He sat down before me, asking his girlfriend to follow. I would have preferred to speak to the patient, but he leaned forward suggestively, telling me that she was having some abnormal discharge, 'I told you about the expiry date condoms, *na*.'

Of course I knew, and so did many other people, but I held that back. I had had enough of him. I firmly asked him to wait outside.

His girlfriend was a pretty girl, a subordinate in his office. There was nothing seriously wrong with her. She had a daughter from a previous marriage. A contraceptive advice was what she needed, as she couldn't quite trust him. I could very well agree with that. She was keen on the insertion of the copper containing intra-uterine devices. It didn't take much time to do that and, with the necessary advice and an instruction leaflet, she was ready to leave. However, the gentleman still had some queries. 'Hey Doctor! I hope she didn't have any infection? No discharge?'

'None. It's just normal.'

'If you want, I can show you.'

I turned, surprised.

'I am carrying a sample in my pocket, just in case!'

He proceeded to withdraw a carefully-wrapped, small, plastic container from his pocket. Yuck! I cringed inwardly before hurriedly telling him that it was not needed. I reminded myself about my solemn vow about not getting irritated.

'If you are so concerned, please use a proper condom,' I said, hoping fervently he would know what was proper.

He looked satisfied and, with relief, I saw him throwing that 'thing' into the bin and leave with his girlfriend. I turned back to call the next patient. She had hardly settled down when the girlfriend appeared again. She wanted to ask something.

'Actually, my friend wants to know how soon does this Copper-T start working.' It was a genuine enough query and I assured her that it starts working immediately. I should have remembered to tell her that.

'You can have fun tonight!' I couldn't resist teasing and immediately cursed my sense of humour. I didn't want to encourage the couple.

Two minutes later, I saw her again hovering outside my door, with the gentleman pointing her to go inside my chamber. I asked the other patient to lie down on the examination table and asked her to come in.

She asked a bit hesitantly, 'What if we do it frequently, as in more number of times?'

'It won't come in the way,' I replied crisply. I knew what she meant. She left, and I hoped it was for good now.

I had finished seeing the other patient when, again, my 'not-to-be-gone-with-the-wind' patient came back, once again propelled inside by her not-so-easily-ignored boyfriend. Thankfully, she waited for the other lady to leave the room before she entered.

'Now what?' I couldn't help sounding a bit exasperated.

'Is it OK if we… well… do it for a long time?' My patience snapped.

'Don't place me in your bedroom with a whistle. I can't be a referee telling you when to start and when to stop. For God's sake, you both are grown-ups, with children. I am no sex guru.'

At any other time, the visual that my imagination was invoking would have thrown me into fits of laughter, but now I simply glared.

'Madam, please don't be angry. Actually, we thought that since we have paid for this, we might as well clear all our doubts. Next time, we will have to pay again.'

Rather than soothing my nerves, this further inflamed them. He was forgetting the phone calls! Did that too come free with the consultation? I slowly counted to ten to regain my composure.

She had the grace to look a little apologetic, and I, a bit embarrassed by my outburst. I recovered my control. She and her obnoxious partner were my patients. I had forgotten that in my irritation.

'Look, don't be anxious. We have discussed the pros and cons. Now forget it and get on with your life. If you have any problem, come again. And please read the information leaflet that has the answers to most of your queries.'

Thankfully, she left but not before leaving me completely drained. I needed a break and decided to meet my friend, Dr Devyani. She was on duty the night before and I wanted to catch her for a cup of coffee before she went home. She was in the duty room and I couldn't help noticing a strange expression on her face. She was tired, about to leave, and before I could say anything, flopped on the bed and announced, 'I am resigning! I don't want to come to the hospital any more. Come to think of it, I don't want to live any more.' Before she could finish, she was gripped by an intense nausea and rushed to the washroom. I simply stared, wondering what the hell was going on! Devyani came out looking better. Was she suffering from morning sickness? I gently asked her if she wanted to discuss. She cried in disgust, 'If I tell you, I will puke again. If I don't, I shall die of misery!' Maybe we just needed to get out of the ward. I grabbed her purse and pulled her towards the café. We both needed something strong. We ordered a hot cappuccino. That brought back some colour to Devyani's face.

Giving her some time to settle down, I decided to pour out my story first. As I went on to tell her about the couple I had just met, I noticed her eyes going rounder and rounder. Ultimately, she let out a choked cry, 'Wait till you hear about mine!' The coffee had relaxed her and she went on to narrate the incidence. Yet she couldn't prevent her distaste from creeping in.

It was past midnight, and with most of the patients settled, Devyani thought of stretching her tired limbs a little. It was always a good thing to rest whenever you got time, on duty. One never knew what was hidden in the dark folds of the mysterious night. She had barely closed her eyes when the nurse rushed in. There was a patient in the casualty.

The patient walked slowly towards the bed, accompanied by a nurse. The nurse was a fresh recruit from Kerala and was an enthusiastic Hindi learner. She gave the patient a wide smile and asked her in an encouraging tone, '*Kya hua, didi? Kitni pregnancy hai?*' ('What happened, sister? How many months are you pregnant?') She thought all patients coming to the gynae casualty were pregnant. However, this was not taken very kindly by the patient. She gave her a rude scowl and literally pushed her away. The poor nurse rushed towards the doctor's duty room.

Devyani calmed her down and went to see the patient. She was sitting rigid on the bed, behaving as if this should have been the last place to be. Well, nobody had forced her to come here! Hospitals were definitely no picnic spots, but then one doesn't come here by choice. Devyani asked her gently, 'What brings you here?' She kept quiet. 'You must be having some problem?' No answer.

'Come on! It's late at night. Something must be wrong so you chose to be here.' Still she kept quiet.

Normally, we never ask leading questions. However, here Devyani was not willing to waste more time on a patient who was too hostile. So, breaking some set of rules, she asked, 'Listen, are you pregnant?' She shook her head. Grateful for the small mercy, Devyani prodded again, 'Are you bleeding?' She again shook her head.

Long duty hours do not leave you with much patience, and Devyani was no exception. Yet, she held on to its fast disappearing vestiges with difficulty.

'Pain? Any burning? Any gynae complain?' She kept on shaking her head in the negative.

Baffled, she was about to ask for her husband or any relative, when her husband came to stand by her side. He probably knew that she was not talking, so he reprimanded her saying, 'Tell her your problem. You are supposed to be frank with the doctor.' The patient looked at the husband with so much wrath that he staggered and asked to wait outside. Devyani had a vague suspicion forming in her head. Sometime back, she had a patient with a retained condom, but she was not throwing tantrums. Whatever the anger of this patient, it was definitely out of proportion.

Through the husband, she came to know that the woman was about thirty-five years old and they had two children, the youngest being about seven years old. He didn't volunteer much after this and preferred waiting outside.

Not knowing what exactly plagued her, Devyani thought of completing the examination and then decide the next course of action. Maybe if the patient still remained un-cooperative, she would have to do some honest talking with the husband. The patient didn't mind going into the examination room at all – rather she went there easily on her own. As she lay down, they could sniff a strange smell in the air. Maybe the staff had eaten something in the labour room (they were quick to deny that!). As she examined her, Devyani noticed something strange, sticky, yet thick in consistency, coming out of her. She recoiled. She had never seen anything like this. A bad infection with such a peculiar odour? Maybe it was a sexually transmitted infection from her partner! That actually explained her anger at the husband. However, before she could linger further, one of the ward *bai* (maid) shouted, 'Ma'am! It looks like a banana!' She was shocked and suddenly the patient sprang up and started crying. Was it really? We all stared as the poor woman, through her hiccups, nodded in affirmative.

Devyani was once again clutching her abdomen, as a fresh round of nausea gripped her. I tried to soothe her, 'You should have pulled out the peel.' Devyani was aghast. 'What the hell are you talking about? There was no peel! I spent one hour cleaning her. All the while, the patient kept crying, feeling just as miserable as us. Her anger and shame were now understandable. Even after all this, the patient didn't speak much. She didn't elaborate on how it all happened and we were repelled enough to not probe the details. As it is, her privacy had been invaded, and we didn't want to hurt her further. With the new insight, we didn't want to talk to her husband at all and sent them both home. The stiffness, the animosity that oozed out of her, somehow felt justified now.' It was now more than five hours, but the pungent odour refused to leave her senses. Devyani was still struggling to forget.

'One thing is very sure. I am off bananas for all my life.' With that, Devyani rushed to the washroom again. And so was I.

I shuddered. Indeed, we were living in the land of *Kamasutra*, seasoned with some shades of grey. Two Mr Greys were enough to be seen in one day in a place as pristine as a hospital.

My wayward thoughts were broken by other doctors joining us at our coffee table. Dr Parul was expecting, and smiled at me as she joined our table. However, to my horror, she took out a banana and started peeling it off. From the corner of my eye, I could see Devyani walking out of the washroom towards our table. 'Devyani, let's get out of here!' I shrieked, and ran towards her before we had to face the startled expression of Parul and all those eyes which had turned towards us. I didn't want Devyani to spend all her day in the washroom!

Phew! We hated bananas.

4
SHADES OF GREY PART II

"Eyes had bared
the moment of folly,
Time to bury once again
an untold story…"

'Doctor! What's wrong with my daughter?'

I turned to an old man who staggered even as he tried to speak authoritatively.

His wife turned her face in disgust. '*Hosh aa gaya aapko? Khyal aa gaya beti ka?*' ('Have you finally come to your senses? Are you finally concerned about your daughter?')

'You keep quiet! You are the one who has spoilt her.'

'That's because I am around her, not you.'

The daughter was temporarily forgotten. She lay bleeding while her parents were busy fixing responsibilities. About time they did that! Shaking my head I said, 'Excuse me, but this is neither the time nor the place.'

Their daughter, a 23-year-old girl, was found lying in a pool of blood in her bedroom, cold and scared to death. Her mother had rushed her to the hospital. She had a thready pulse and low blood pressure. The emergency team tried to resuscitate her even as they struggled with the antecedent cause. To our shock, she was found bleeding profusely, vaginally. This mystery was getting thicker than the fog outside. Was it a sexual assault or rape? The girl was conscious enough to know what was going on. She looked surprised at the mention of rape. She shook her head wildly and struggled to say, 'The door!', but before she could speak any further, she started sinking again. She was losing blood faster than we were giving her. Nobody was forthcoming, and nothing explained her predicament. Whatever the precipitating factor, it was more important to stop the bleeding. The word was spreading around much to the discomfort of the still squabbling parents. We had to shift her fast to the operation theatre, away from the avid glances of the curious onlookers.

The mother howled, collapsing her weight over her relatives, unmindful of their groan. 'She was home. She never went out, neither did anyone come to our place. I swear! We just had dinner, and I was watching television while she went to her room.' Her father smirked and scoffed. The relatives tried to act smart. 'Why are the doctors not able to tell us anything? These days, they don't understand much until they get expensive tests done, and empty your pockets.'

This was really without any provocation, and our patience snapped. 'She was found bleeding at home! Can you explain how it happened?' That put them in the spot. Maybe they had come to the hospital just to create trouble. Ungracious people! Then I thought of life draining out of the poor girl slowly, and I knew where my priorities lay. I rushed towards the operation theatre.

The girl had been brought in suspicious circumstances. Maybe we should inform the police.

She was about to be shifted inside for surgery when the ward boy came running. She wanted to talk to me before she was put under anaesthesia. She was almost breathless and barely managed to whisper, 'Madam, please don't report to the police. It's not rape, I swear! I hurt myself.'

There was something convincing about her. Maybe she had indeed fallen down.

'The door handle!' She was too weak to elaborate further, and without wasting much time, we shifted her to the theatre. We had more pertinent issues to worry about.

Under anaesthesia, one could finally make some sense of what was going on. Fresh blood could be seen gushing down from inside her vagina. As we struggled to catch the offending bleeders, to our horror, we discovered a deep laceration extending into the deepest recess of her vagina. Along with it, the cervix, which was the outer opening of her uterus (womb), was torn grievously and gaped at us. Just a thin rim of tissue was keeping it precariously attached to the parent body, bleeding and hanging loose, making it look almost like a bucket handle. Was she actually hiding a serious assault? This looked more like an injury with a sharp object. A little to the front, and her urinary bladder would have gone; a little behind, and her rectum or bowel would have been injured. The girl had a miraculous escape! Her tissue had become friable, and it was sheer patience and grit that saw us through. We finally managed to put some order to the traumatised tissues, and control the bleeders.

Her secrets were threatening to spill all over. She was hiding something for sure. We waited for her to come to her senses. The girl had a lot to explain.

Outside, we were greeted by hostile relatives. An unmarried girl with an unexplained injury; there was always a stigma attached. It was better to refrain from speaking much to them. Her father, who had not yet sobered, still wanted to know how it all happened. He was irritating us, but we realized that he meant to blame and irritate his wife more. Their otherwise intolerable domestic squabbles would have lightened up the tense atmosphere had it not been for the cloud of suspicion hanging around their daughter.

She was doing well, and leaving her in the post-operative ward, I went back to my clinic. A young woman, looking serene, with a shawl draped carefully over her head, was waiting for me. She followed me inside.

'Doctor, I keep having urine infections off and on.'

She looked at me for a moment. I guessed there was more to come, but she probably thought otherwise and kept quiet. A little bit of infection was all I could see. As I sat down to write down medicines, she blurted out, 'I am guilty, doctor! I have done things I am not proud of.'

'Aren't we all? Nothing unusual about that, dear.' I tried to make things light for her.

'Actually my husband, you know… he doesn't understand my needs. He only thinks about himself.' She was almost in tears.

'Have you ever tried speaking to him?'

'I have, on many occasions. But he looks baffled. According to him, he does everything to make me happy – from buying clothes and jewellery, to taking me on expensive holidays… He thinks we have a wonderful sex life too,' she added, bitterly. Obviously, they did not.

'I think you need to be more honest.'

'I have been blunt, at times. But he's over and done with, even before I can talk to him. He is only bothered about himself. It's all about my duty, not his. You know how husbands are!'

Did I? She sounded sure, so maybe I did, I thought humorously.

Now what was she guilty about? A secret boyfriend, I wondered! Was my clinic a confession box, today? Sometimes it did help talking to strangers and getting that load off your head. I couldn't deny her that.

'I can't depend on him. He has failed me. I use other "things" to satisfy myself. Maybe that's why I keep having infections. One day, I know I will have cancer and I will pay for my sins.' There was a fresh bout of tears.

I wondered who was teaching her these things. Maybe another equally ill-informed friend.

'You have not committed any sin. It's really all right. Don't worry much.' So many taboos we suffer unnecessarily from!

The façade of a happy married life was fast slipping, showing a suffering wife and a husband whose vanity made him so selfish and ignorant. Luckily for him, she didn't turn to a boyfriend.

'A boyfriend will complicate things,' she said, as if she could read my mind.

I tried to counsel her. Maybe they both needed to sit down and do some honest talking. About time he accepted that it was not only about men, but about women too. Equality in the bedroom! I could see a new gender equation coming up.

And if he was not forthcoming, then maybe she could carry on without feeling guilty. She left, promising to come again next week, with reports.

My phone beeped again and I was informed that our visitor in the post-operative ward had woken up and wanted to talk.

She was lying quietly in her bed. The blood transfusions had brought some color back to her face. She looked much relaxed, but a trace of anxiety still marred her features. I waited for her to speak. She started haltingly, 'It wasn't rape.' I listened. That didn't explain her injuries though.

'Actually, I injured myself.'

'You fell down?' Startled, she shook her head again. I was getting confused.

Suddenly she blurted out, 'It was the door handle.' I remembered her saying something about a door handle before she was shifted to the operation theatre. Where was this leading to?

'You fell over it?' The torn cervix, like a 'bucket handle' as we fancifully called it, loomed large in my vision. How on earth could a fall over a door cause such a terrible injury?

'I inserted it!' she blurted out. Did she really mean that? I looked at her, horrified.

'Why on earth did you do that?' I said, before I could stop myself.

I was reminded of another girl I had seen some time back. She was an unmarried girl who kept us guessing till she came to the point. She ultimately admitted that all she could think of was somebody 'digging, digging' all the time. The feeling was so strong that it almost consumed her.

'If guys can do it, why can't I?' she replied defensively, breaking my train of thoughts.

Exactly! 'Why should boys have all the fun?' my favourite heroine Priyanka Chopra whispered in my ears, as she smoothly rode her pink scooty. Yes, why indeed? Gender equality once again! A female trying to restore the gender balance in her own queer way. For a long time, I was at a loss for words as I tried to come to terms with her justification.

'My dear, do you realize how dangerous your little game could have been? You were just short of injuring your bladder and bowel, not to mention the mess you made of your uterus.'

If she was scared she didn't show it. There was a tinge of defiance creeping in. 'My boyfriend flaunts too much. I was fed up of his taunts. I wanted to be sure everything was fine with me.' This was getting weird. It was any day more sensible to dump the insensitive boyfriend. She did have a lot to sort out, I guess. She looked tired, and as she lay with her head bent towards one side, I couldn't help but empathize with her.

'Please don't tell my parents anything' she pleaded.

Culture imposes certain rules, but then people have desires. Desire breaks all rules. Desperate desires, desperate situations!

I was met outside by her scowling father who was still restless to know the exact sequence of events.

'Your daughter has woken up. She says that she had fallen and injured herself' was all that was told to him.

He stared disbelievingly, demanding more. 'How could she? Can that cause so much bleeding?'

'You need to ask her that. And yes, injuries there can bleed a lot.'

Her mother, who was looking quite grim, stood quiet. I wish I could ask them if the doors in their house were not very old and the handles not rusted. Thank God for the tetanus shots we gave her pre-operatively.

However, I walked away before giving in to the temptation of discussing the furniture at their place. I simply didn't want to know anything about a broken handle!

My day had just begun. I had so much more to discover. I had just opened my eyes.

Streaks of grey clouds were marring the bright horizon overhead. Shades of grey! It thundered. Soon, we would have respite from the searing heat. I knew it was going to rain ...

5
THE URCHIN'S DREAM

"From a drunken man's desire
To a shrunken man's ire,
A reluctant prey
To the damning fire!
She had lived it all
But then life moved on…"

The outdoor gynaecology clinic in a government hospital is not something to look forward to, especially after a busy duty the night before. However, it is here that you really comprehend how fast the population of India is growing, and also how most women are obsessed with one organ of their body – the mysterious womb, or the uterus! Everything they suffer is somehow related to it. From something as vague as a simple backache, to something as weird as mood changes, it's always because of that. You also see the extremes of life here. From one woman desperate to get pregnant, to the next one waiting to get rid of her baby fast enough, it's all here. As a first-year postgraduate, I often wondered if our sexuality was indeed our nemesis! But then, it is here that you meet the most self sacrificing, and the most loving of God's creations – yes, we call them women!

We made our way with difficulty through the noisy corridors, lined with those waiting for their turn. People love to engage in animated conversations, even outside a doctor's clinic! It was somehow difficult to manage those engrossed in deep gossip. Once settled, we started summoning them individually, asking men to stay out. However, as it transpired, most patients took inexplicable pride in not understanding anything. They listened to the doctor with a blank expression before requesting them to repeat it all to their respective husbands or mothers-in-law, who, according to them, were probably the most intelligent people in the world. Looking back, I think it was a smart move on their part to put all accountability on someone else. The older women generally looked at the young doctors with disdain. '*Inko kya samajh mein ayega?*' ('What'll they understand?') One pregnancy, one child, and they were a better obstetrician and peadiatrician.

Anyway, patience and tolerance is an art you learn gradually, as I was slowly discovering.

As I looked around, I noticed a small, thin, and dark woman with unkempt, short hair, wearing a dirty shirt and torn pants. I could have easily missed her for a boy. Remembering my visit to the mental asylum few days back, where I saw women getting their hair chopped like this, I grimaced, 'Maybe another one!'

The nurse called out 'Shahana!' Without raising my head, I could see somebody sitting on the stool next to me. Arrogance is something which is not in short supply, even in places such as hospitals and I must admit I was not left untouched by it. It made me forgo the finer nuances of extending a formal greeting to those we called 'patients'.

'*Kya problem hai?*' ('What's the problem?')

'Good morning, ma'am!'

I was surprised to listen to this. Feeling guilty and suddenly remembering my manners I said, 'Good morning!' As I raised my head, I saw the same dirty, street urchin kind of woman sitting next to me.

Hiding my surprise at her smart tone, I asked again, '*Jaldi bolo, kya problem hai?*' ('Tell me quickly, what's your problem?')

She said, 'I want to get pregnant.'

'Are you married?' I asked before I could stop myself. If she was surprised, she didn't show it.

'Yes! I have been married for about four months. My husband is an autorickshaw driver,' she said.

'It is not a very long time to be married, and you should wait for a few more months before coming to us,' I advised her.

Suddenly, she started pleading, 'Ma'am, I may not live very long and I want to give something to my husband and my mother-in-law who love me so much.'

Suddenly full of intrigue, I couldn't help asking her the reason. She silently took out a paper and I realised that sitting in front of me was a 25-year-old HIV-positive woman.

'Do you realize the problems you and your unborn child can have?'

She remained adamant.

'Have you ever been pregnant before?' I asked.

'Many times! But I always got an abortion,' she replied.

There was something strange going on and I had to get to the bottom of this. After taking a detailed history, I took her inside the examining room. And there, to my disgust, I pulled out a T-shaped device from inside her.

Do you know what this is? If you want to get pregnant, why did you get this Copper-T inserted?' I wondered who had put this, as it was not common to put these intrauterine devices in women who didn't have any children.

Seeing that, she broke into tears. 'I don't know much about this, ma'am.'

Silent sobs shook her body as she cried helplessly. I took her back to my chamber and got a glass of water for her. I asked her to calmly tell me all about it. And what came out shocked the hell out of me ...

Shahana was from Bangalore. Life was pretty all right till she lost her mother at the age of ten. Her father was a brutal man. Drunk most of the time, he spent his time, and whatever money he earned as a rickshaw puller, on cheap whiskey and women. She was a good student, and inspite of all, managed to keep going to her school. She suffered his unprovoked beating and verbal abuse as she didn't have much choice. And then one day, he brought her some very nice clothes and sweets. She had turned fifteen that day. Happy to see some sign of affection from her father and eager to please him, she went and changed. Suddenly, he entered her room and told her that he was very short of money, and as his daughter, she had some duties towards him. She was his only source of income and he had sold her for fifty thousand rupees. She drew back, shocked. How could he? She begged him to keep her with him. She promised to earn by doing any menial job. However, he grew angry. Warning her, he went outside and came back drunk, late at night. She decided to plead with him one more time, but when she went to his room, he was in a very different mood...

Suddenly, she could not continue telling me any longer and started sobbing. It was the darkest night of her life. The protector turned out to be her destroyer, and she lost all that she had, that day. It was not only her body, but also her soul that was raped. She went numb with shame and grief. She lived in a dumb stupor for a few days before, one day, a man came to take her away.

She was kept at many shabby places, and life went on getting murkier. She lived in such dungeons for some years, never quiet accepting what life had made her out to be. She also discovered that she conceived very easily. She had multiple abortions and, once, she was told that there was a T-shaped device that could prevent pregnancies. Her madam insisted, and it was put inside her after one such abortion. The next few years did not see any conception but the disgust with herself steadily grew, and so did the determination to break free.

One evening, on the pretext of going to the weekly bazaar, she crept out of the brothel and escaped. She reached a hair dresser's shop and chopped off her hair. She changed into an old shirt and pants, to escape recognition. After that, she reached the railway station. A train stationed there was going to Delhi. She boarded it, without knowing her destination. She could hardly sleep, scared of being caught. At the Gwalior station, she got down for some food. Before she could climb back, the train had started moving and she was left at the station. Most people took her for a dirty, teenaged boy and did not spare any glance. Getting bolder, she ventured out of the station. However, the events of the past few days had left her feeing giddy. She remembered seeing an autorickshaw stopping in front of her before she lost her senses and passed out.

When she woke up, she saw an old woman gently kneeling over her. She was wiping her head, and as soon as she woke up, the woman shouted for her son, 'Hey look, Shyam! She is awake.' Shyam rushed in and she could see them relax.

'Are you all right?' he asked her sympathetically. 'Who are you and where were you coming from?' She kept quiet. 'It's all right. We will not force you to tell us anything. But you need to eat something. I am sorry, I took you for a boy.' He looked sheepish. 'I thought you were someone who had run away from home. I wanted to take you back once you were awake. But when I reached home, mother scolded me for bringing a woman. I am sorry. I didn't mean to hurt you.' She still kept quiet, though at heart, she marvelled at their generosity. She never knew such people existed.

They insisted that she stay with them till she was better. Gradually, she settled in their house. For the first time in her life, she felt safe and happy. Shyam's mother showered her with maternal affection. Shyam mostly kept quiet, but she could feel his silent admiration many a time. Scarred by her past, she did not dare encourage him. One day, his mother proposed to her that she marry her son. She was speechless. Was it really happiness knocking her doors, finally? It was then that she told them her whole story. When she finished, Shyam's mother clasped her tightly in her arms, while he stood silent, anger and hatred for her tormentors reflected in his eyes, and his fists clenched.

She got married to him a few days later, but her happiness was short lived as she started falling sick quiet often. She was diagnosed as being HIV-positive. However, even during her illness, knowing well the stigma attached with the disease, her husband and his mother remained her pillars of support. So she now wanted to pay them back with the only thing that she could – a baby. She had really forgotten about that Copper T. She thanked me repeatedly for removing that.

I couldn't help asking about her mother-in-law and husband. It is ironical that people who are not so privileged sometimes do things bolder and wiser than their more privileged counterparts. She proudly called for them. Her husband entered the chamber shyly, along with his mother. They simply folded their hands in gratitude. And I, who all this while thought that my degree had somehow made me more superior, felt small and inconspicuous in front of such fearless and selfless people. Moved beyond speech, I bowed and folded my hands quietly, before quickly writing down some tests and medicines for Shahana. I had a herculean job ahead now. I had to help her pay back her debts. Somehow, those few minutes that I spent with her had changed a lot of things. It had earned her more respect and dignity, and me, more humility.

As quietly as they had come, they moved out of the clinic. Taking a deep breath, I called for the next patient. Life had to move on...

6
THE UNEXPECTED VISITOR

"While the word slumbers in sleep,
Labouring she struggles.
A hand rouses from deep,
Even while it cuts to relieve
a scar it will always leave…"

The impatient ringing of the telephone interrupted my brief sojourn. My sleep-deprived eyes looked at the phone, praying for it to not be another emergency.

'Hello!'

The cheerful voice from the other side pleased my dulled-out senses. It was my friend who was on duty on the surgical side. Half of the girls of our hostel would have given anything to swap places with me to listen to his voice in the middle of the night. It brought a reluctant smile.

'Hello! What brings you to our labour room?'

'Oh well, I am told that the hot RMO (Resident Medical Officer) is on duty today. The one from Bhopal.'

I could hear his naughty grin but I was in no mood for silly gibberish at this time, 'Cut it out and tell me fast.'

We residents had this knack of reading the tired minds of others on duty. Labour room duty in a government hospital was not a picnic. Rather, it was a waterloo for the easily fatigued ones. Maybe my friend sensed my agitated state and replied, 'Oh well, I have a gift for you. Sending her fast. Do get back to me. Best of luck!'

Abruptly, the phone went quiet. Irritated by him for not divulging any details, I decided to not get back to him at all.

Without giving me much time to ponder, a girl still in her school uniform – a white shirt and a crumpled blue skirt, with her hair plaited in red ribbons – walked inside, holding her father's hand.

'*Arre baba, bahar ruko* (Hey, please wait outside),' our nurse shouted at the father.

Her father stopped, looking worried. The girl, tensing slightly, held on to his hand even more firmly. There was something about her that made me say, 'You stay in the casualty room. I will see you there.'

Leaving the labour room, I took them to the examination room.

'Sit down and tell me your problem.'

Still holding the hand of her father, she sat there quietly. I kept asking her but she didn't reply.

Her father folded his hands and pleaded, 'Doctor *sahib*, my daughter is in a lot of pain, since yesterday. We tried everything in the village but to no avail. I left my village at 9 am and have been going places in this hospital. Everyone says she is not our case.'

I was about to say that she didn't look more than twelve, not likely to be a gynae case either, but something made me stay quiet. Maybe it was the anguish in her eyes, the slight tremble of her hands as she clutched on to her father, or the visible lump in her abdomen. She could be a case of those rare ovarian tumours of childhood. I speculated silently. They do twist and cause lot of pain. However, more than pain I could see fear lurking in her eyes. There was nothing unusual about it; kids were often scared of hospitals. With a lot of coaxing and a little reprimand, I managed to make the girl let go of her father's hand and lie on the examination table.

What I saw, startled me. The little girl was a case of full term pregnancy with labour pains, or rather having strong contractions with very little time left. In fact, she was just about to deliver! A little late and she would have easily made a spectacle of herself on the roads. As we rushed her into the delivery room, I marvelled at her endurance. Any other woman would have brought the ward down with her screams, but here this girl was silently holding her father's hand all the while. It's really an amazing world. Maybe that's the reason it is said that pain is always in the mind.

Her father, despite our angry outbursts and persistence, feigned ignorance of her pregnant state. The girl, as expected, was just not talking. Neither of them answered any of our questions. Her father just kept his hands folded all the time. Not wanting to waste much time, I moved to her side. As she lay down on the labour table, the other women next to her let out shrill cries.

'Don't howl! Look at her. She is so much younger than all of you and is tolerating her pains so well,' our senior nurse scolded them.

Most of them stopped screaming, in astonishment. For most women, labour was a celebration, preceded by nine months of indulgence by their families. Nurtured with care and affection, they looked forward to this day. On this day, it was not a baby, but a mother, who was born.

Unaware of the turmoil going on in the minds of the others, the girl needed little help and delivered smoothly, without any fuss. She even allowed us to suture her much to the surprise of the whole labour room staff that had gathered around. Was she in some kind of shock, or was it nature at its primitive best? Maybe she was hiding something. Whatever it was, she became a role model for other labouring women. They became quieter and well behaved. The moment we were through with her, like a child she jumped down from the labour table, unmindful of her stitches. Ignoring our warnings, she started walking, asking for her father. She refused to acknowledge the baby, and there was no flicker of any emotion betraying her having undergone so much pain just minutes before.

Nights in the hospitals generally stand still with a quiet elegance. The frenzy of the day softly gives way to an eerie silence, as if the hospital heals to brave once again the pain, suffering and anguish of the next day. But the silence of that night was broken by hurried footsteps and noisy phone calls. The news had spread like fire. There were repeated calls and enquiries from people willing to adopt the baby. The girl could not be entrusted with the baby, and her father had gone out. The staff was given clear instructions to keep the baby safe and secure. The hospital could not participate in any undercover dealing between the family and people wanting to adopt the baby. And if they abandoned it, we had to inform the police and hand over the baby to government institutes. I entrusted our senior nurses to take care of the neonate.

While we were busy, the reluctant mother had quietly vanished from the labour room. That led to another round of frenzy. She was soon found sitting outside the labour room with her father, enjoying a cup of tea and a hot samosa.

The baby was a healthy boy. The nurses enjoyed looking after him. The night was almost over and the father now wanted to go home with his daughter. They didn't wish to stay back. Till then the hospital staff were busy tackling couples desperate to take the baby. It was an effort warding off all the calls, and security guards were deployed outside the hospital to prevent any mishap.

Of those who thronged to the hospital, some had been married for over ten years, tried for pregnancy long enough before accepting that they could never have a biological child. Faced with endless queues and long wait at the orphanages, they were desperate enough to take the baby at any cost. I often wondered if God was really fair. On what basis did he deprive some and keep burdening others? What *karmas* (deeds) had this baby committed to be abandoned by his own parents? Was the *karma* of his past birth catching up, or was God planning something adventurous for the baby? Whichever way, one could never understand the workings of the Almighty. He knew the best.

The father and the girl approached me once again. They wanted to leave. I tried hard to know more about the girl and the events preceding the delivery, but the father remained adamant on his stand of not knowing anything about it. And for all the time that she was with us, the girl refused to talk. I had seen parents going into blind rage once they got to know about the pregnancy of their unmarried daughter, but here the father maintained his composure. I doubted his ignorance. Was it a result of rape, or incest? I refused to consider, even for a moment, for it to be consensual at her age. Did that explain her strange behaviour? Considering her age, it was pertinent to inform the police.

The father insisted that she was eighteen. Maybe he anticipated trouble, for before we could get them to sign the papers and complete the formalities, the father-daughter duo left. They disappeared with the baby, none of them betraying the scars of the night before. I marvelled at the selfishness of human beings. I had seen people breaking down if something went wrong with their baby. And here, without any remorse, the mother was ready to sacrifice her baby. Probably she was not old enough to understand the gravity of the situation.

It was time for me also, to call it a day. The excitement of the night was catching up. I called up my surgeon friend and told him about the patient he had referred. He was amazed and told me that the casualty officer had taken her case for an abdominal tumor and sent the patient to them, adding that he knew it was pregnancy as soon as he saw her. But even he had not expected her to be in such an advanced stage of labour.

As I was about to leave, one of our staff came rushing towards me. 'Ma'am, do you know they went to the bus stand? They have given the baby to a couple.'

'Do you know them?' I asked her.

She looked slightly uncomfortable and avoided looking at me. I didn't prompt much as I didn't want to be part of any controversy. 'I hope they paid her something,' I mumbled to myself.

She replied quickly, 'Of course ma'am! They paid for their tickets, gave five hundred rupees to them and also one hundred for some *chai-nashta* (tea and biscuits)' she boasted of their generosity. 'The couple belong to a rich business family and would keep the baby well.'

The greed and selfishness of the act amazed me. I was filled with a strange regret and a sense of unfairness for the girl. 'I am sure they know how to do business,' I replied sarcastically.

What a strange world we live in. When we don't have something, we are ready to go to any lengths for it. However, when it comes within our reach, we start being all practical and rational. For God's sake! They had got a child! They should have given some consideration to the woman who had risked her life for them, even though not by choice. As for the girl and her father, I was sure they would have been relieved. They couldn't wait enough to be rid of the unwanted baggage and must have been thankful for even those five hundred rupees. How selfish and mean, circumstances make us. And the baby! Disowned by his biological family and grabbed by his adoptive parents who chanced upon this God-sent opportunity, would they ever tell him that he was abandoned by his mother near the state roadways bus stand? Probably he would he never get to know the real story of his birth. Maybe it was better this way, than be with a mother who could never talk about his parentage. As Shakespeare had said, 'All's well that ends well'.

The dust and heat in the city was rising and it was time for me to go home. The father-daughter duo must have crossed the city borders by now. I could almost visualize her resting her head firmly on her father's shoulders, her hands tucked securely in his, as they disappeared into anonymity. I hoped her young mind would wipe out whatever it was holding on to, and one day she would be free of her past.

However, a little girl in her crumpled school uniform and red ribbons would keep knocking at my conscience for a long time. The memories of my unexpected visitor were going to linger forever…

7
THE WIDOW

"Behind a veil of tradition,
And some unholy conventions,
The deeds of past breathe free.
Raising its ugly head,
Scorned the moral brigade.
For a woman had sinned,
She had dared to shock!
And life faltered,
Stood aghast…"

A silent corner stood forlorn in the labour ward. The air around it hung with remembered pain and suffering. A final checkpoint before a tragedy, that loomed large, unraveled itself. It had a brooding quality about it, and even when unoccupied, looked forbidding. It was called 'the septic labour room'. I often shivered when I crossed it during my night rounds. There were a few places in the hospital which were actually spooky. This included the burns ward, the eclampsia room, and the septic labour room.

They were shrouded with haunted tales. The senior staff and
nurses particularly relished narrating them. Maybe they knew
that it got under our skin. There is undoubtedly always a strange
fascination about ghost stories. From the story of Kamla Raja in
her famous white dress walking the central quadrangle for her
midnight rendezvous, to the anguished cries coming from the
burns ward and the creaking doors of the septic labour room, you
were hooked to them. Most of them were fabricated, by-products
of a fertile imagination. The tormented souls would know better
than to walk with us present day humans, but try as I might,
I couldn't shrug off these nocturnal visitors from my mind.
Whenever I walked the silent corridors of a watchful hospital at
night, I would subconsciously look for them. Very unbecoming of
a doctor who has seen death at such close quarters!

The occupants of the septic room were unfortunate patients
who suffered serious infections during pregnancy. Apart from
jaundice, we very frequently saw cases of septic abortions
admitted there. Septic abortions were the result of abortions done
in an improper way resulting in fatal infections, usually carried
out by an unqualified person. In the days before the MTP Act
(Medical Termination of Pregnancy Act) came into force in
1971, it was a leading cause of death amongst pregnant woman.
The Act had strict provisions. It clearly set out the conditions
as to when abortions could be done, the place where they could
be done, and the people who could perform it. Yet decades
later, in a country where ignorance is deadlier than a disease, it
continued to kill unsuspecting and vulnerable women rampantly.
The majority of them were unmarried girls, widows, or victims of
incest. Hiding behind a veil of tradition and lack of confidence in
modern medicine, people still resorted to unscrupulous quacks.
Probably it was the secrecy they provided…

However, for some chauvinistic men, abortion still remained
a method of contraception, a routine in a woman's life that
hardly needed much thought. The present day Shah Jahan can
hardly afford to build a Taj Mahal for his wife, yet he doesn't

mend his ways. It is guilt that casts a shadow over the opulence of the monument. Beyond its beautiful exteriors, the Taj Mahal breathes the poignant tale of Mumtaz Mahal who died during her fourteenth childbirth. In his days, Shah Jahan didn't have much choice. Now we have so much more, but women still die due to ignorance, and sometimes even due to the insolence of their partners.

A group engaged in a heated discussion suddenly became quiet as I approached them. I could sense there was something wrong from their troubled voices and grave expressions. A woman draped in a saree, with a dupatta tied over her forehead, was sitting with them. As I drew close, the crowd dispersed, leaving the woman with only a few relatives there. As she raised her flushed head I could see a tinge of fear clouding her eyes. I recoiled as I touched her. She was burning hot! There was a pungent odour all around. Sometimes, these patients travelled a long distance covered in blankets and it was not very unusual for them to carry that smell.

'What's wrong with you?' I asked her gently.

'Madam, she has been having fever for the last five days. It is not going down despite medicines,' a woman, who had accompanied her, replied before she could answer. The patient looked dazed.

I looked around for her husband. There were certain things he needed to answer, if she was not talking.

'She was widowed a year back. She has no children either,' the relative told me, as if sensing what I wanted to know.

'Is there any possibility that she might have conceived?'

'We told you ma'am, she is a widow,' a female relative who looked much older, and was probably her mother-in-law, reminded me sternly. I ignored her and asked the relatives to wait outside.

It was important to rule out pregnancy before we started any treatment.

'OK, you can tell me now. Are you overdue?'

She shook her head. Even alone, she was emphatic in her denial and didn't reveal much. Sighing, I went on with my examination. I could see purulent discharge coming out and her uterus appeared to be a little bulky and tender. I took the swabs for culture. Maybe this could be a bad pelvic infection? She was stable, even though her pulse was running fast. She kept on licking her dry, cracked lips, pointing towards her dehydrated state. I flicked through her previous reports. It was her ultrasound that caught my attention. It was suggestive of retained products of conception. So was I seeing a septic abortion despite the reluctance of the patient to admit even a remote pregnancy. No wonder there was so much emphasis on her widowed status. I had no idea of what had transpired before she came to us. My only connection with her past was this report. Very firmly, the implication of her ultrasound report was explained to her, but how could one corroborate the ultrasound finding if she gave no history of abortion, spontaneous or induced?

'Listen, don't be scared. Tell me what happened?' I prodded again. She simply refused to budge. I was rattled by her irrational behaviour. I fervently hoped to speak to her parents. Sometimes, parents are more forthcoming and concerned but, sadly, they were still on the way.

'Doctor *saab*, what's wrong with her?' her relatives entered and wanted to know. They were hiding facts, yet expected the doctors to tell them the exact diagnosis.

'We suspect septic abortion.'

I could sense their hostility and immediate withdrawal,

'She is a widow! Do you want to ostracize us?'

My patience wavered, and threatened to snap. In a fraction of a second, the 'concerned' relatives were gone and, in their place, sneered the moral brigade. Did a doctor have any say in that? They didn't have any inkling of the danger she was in.

'She has a high risk of going into septicemia and dying. If you don't trust us, you are free to take her anywhere.' That put them in a tight spot. With apparent misgivings, they complied and got her admitted. The septic labour room was inhabited once again. This time, a young 28-year-old woman, hiding behind a cloak of secrecy and a past, demanding redemptions.

She was put on broad-spectrum, high antibiotics, but in vain. Little did we know about the deadly focus of infection she was still carrying. Rather than improving, her condition started deteriorating rapidly. Her cultures showed a definite growth of bacteria. The fever refused to break down and, to top it all, her intestines stopped moving. She was fast developing peritonitis (an infection of the abdomen) and intestinal obstruction. A repeat ultrasound pointed to something suspicious inside the uterus. A perforation of the uterus and a gut injury were suspected. The situation was akin to swinging between Scylla and Charybdis. Taking note of her lack of improvement, with an obvious foci of infection, surgery was warranted. However, it was heroic to operate in the setting of sepsis. In spite of the gravity of the situation, the relatives became scarce and remained in a permanent state of denial. Her elder brother-in-law was often seen hovering around her. An informed consent about her life-threatening condition and need for surgery was sought with difficulty, and after much deliberation, the patient was taken up for surgery.

The surgery itself was no less of a marathon. We had to remove the offending structure from the uterus. One didn't have to do much. The object of suspicion soon popped into my hand. Much to the revulsion of everyone, it was a ragged broomstick! Somebody must have put some medicine on it and inserted it inside the uterus for abortion. Her fetid abdomen further shocked our senses. The whole gut had turned putrid – almost green. None of us had ever heard or seen something so gruesome. A woman deserved, at least, some dignity. How horrid must have been the person who put it there! And why were they all so tight-lipped about the whole thing? Who were they protecting so fiercely? Even the most mercenary doctor would never do this vile act. It had to be the handiwork of some mean and outrageous quack. Was it a glorified *dai*, or some malicious *tantric* (shaman)?

There were government hospitals offering treatment free of cost everywhere. There must be something terribly wrong in our system that people choose to come here only towards the end.

The surgical team was called in. Meanwhile, we had to explain to the attendants her condition and her poor prognosis, which meant another confrontation with them. There was only her anxious brother-in-law pacing outside the operation theatre.

'This is what we found inside her.' I pointed towards the tray containing the offending broomstick. Startled, as if caught red-handed, he looked back at me. I could see he was worried. However, he quickly regained his composure.

'We know nothing about this.' He lowered his eyes.

'Someone must have put it there? Did you take her to a *dai*?' I persisted. For reasons best known to him, he chose not to answer that. Surprisingly, he did not charge back, probably warned by the contemptuous look in my eyes. However, even in the face of such daring evidence, not much was forthcoming from him. Feeling like banging my head against a wall, I went back. Her intestines had been resected and a colostomy (an opening of the bowel directly to the skin) made. The stench coming from her abdomen hung in the operation theatre, a poignant reminder of the unforgiving saga. The woman remained critical, and once the surgery was over, she was shifted to the ICU. She was toxic with a resistant infection, but strangely, she remained conscious and well-oriented.

I, a young ambitious doctor, early in my post-graduate days, dreamt of changing the society. I nursed notions that the bad would one day be exposed and punished, and truth shall finally triumph. However, as they say, time is the biggest teacher. Something inside me had rebelled at this blatant abuse of a woman. She might have sinned in the eyes of her family, but there was no logic behind the injustice meted out to her.

I got determined to get to the bottom of this and find out the person behind this ghastly episode. My matrons and senior colleagues mocked me. They tried to convince me about the futility of my efforts. 'They just never tell,' would be their standard reply. These things were very common in villages. As it is she was a widow. Even if she died, her family would be relieved. I didn't know her personally, but it hurt me to even think like that. It had become almost an obsession for me. Her resilience made me more persistent. I waited for the façade to break.

'Tell me! I will not breathe a word to any living soul.' She stuck to her silence, despite my reassurances.

'Don't you realize that it is your duty as well to punish this person so that he doesn't destroy any other life?' She just flickered her eyelashes but didn't utter a single word. The cloak of secrecy refused to slip.

I fretted and fumed at the injustice. It was now three days after her surgery, yet she was not improving. Could she really not see reason? On the fourth day, I was told that she was deteriorating. I almost decided not to see her, but my irrational fascination with her once again pushed me to her side.

I was surprised to see her parents outside the ICU. However, my hopes were quashed when they folded their hands and said, 'Madam, you live in the city. Please do not destroy our reputation.'

I was aghast. 'How did we become the culprits? Why aren't you angry at those who endangered your daughter's life?'

They had no answers.

I now realized why doctors were wary of working in rural areas. You could never get past their deep-rooted superstitions and traditions. They were ready to destroy the hospitals and beat up the doctors even if something unintentionally went wrong, but nothing could shake their belief of their own orthodox methods. Quacks flourished fearlessly under the 'watchful' eyes of the law. These unqualified people were the first contact point in the case of most maladies and had made a mockery of modern medicine and the legal system. Even the health agencies were forced to acknowledge this, helpless in the face of the blind faith people had in them.

Reining in my turmoil, I reached by her side. She was, by now, familiar with me. However, today she looked a little disoriented. Her kidneys had stopped working and her breathing was also not getting better. She was developing multiple organ failure, secondary to her septicemia. The ICU people had stabilized her momentarily, but her chances were getting dim. I spoke to her softly, 'This may be the last time we are talking. Please tell me who did this to you. I promise not to harm your family.' She kept quiet but I could see her quiver. I clasped her hands.

I asked her something that was nagging me for a long time. 'Was it someone from the family?' A tiny drop rolled down her cheeks. Somehow, I knew who he was. 'Did he take you to someone for the abortion?'

She clasped my hand strongly. I winced in pain. I knew what she meant. Suddenly, she whispered. She was almost breathless with the effort, 'Please, you won't tell this to anyone.' I promised her, but I needed to know more, 'Who was it? Tell me the name!'

Her skin had become parched with the unremitting fever. 'I don't know,' she sighed.

'Don't you want to punish that person? Haven't you suffered enough?'

She looked at me helplessly, 'I can't. He will kill us.' Tears clouded her eyes and she sobbed. Her truth was as deafening as her silence.

I felt helpless as I couldn't do anything. At least I knew he was a man. However, beyond that I was clueless. Even the fear of an impending death could not break through the wall of dread and fear that she had erected around her. I could do nothing other than be a mute spectator to her grief.

The hypocrisy of the whole system stood stark in the revelation. I stayed with her for some more time. Destiny had already made up its mind on her. I finished my work and left for home. Next day, I was told that she had collapsed and could not be resuscitated. The fatal moment was inevitable. A door had been left ajar by her, deliberately. Her end had walked in, gloating, abetted by an unscrupulous mind. I am sure her family must have been relieved of the baggage they were carrying. They could now bury her with respect. Even in her death, she had not let them down.

However, somewhere in my mind, a pair of dark eyes taunted me mercilessly. I couldn't let go of a cruel mystery man not very far from me, who, undeterred, was inserting broomsticks into women, defying every norm of a civilized society. A young woman died, victim to not only her own helplessness, but to apathetic parents who gave up on their daughter after her marriage, to her family which failed to protect her, a condemned widowhood that didn't look for resettlement but worked undercover with secret alliances and then sought sinister tribulations, and a society that believed women were the sole harbingers of morality and good behaviour. And, above all, an empowered woman, a doctor, who watched helplessly as a young patient died painfully, but surely, in front of her eyes.

I had kept my promise and never breathed a word to her family. Disgust was a mild word for such heinous crimes, majority of which tend to go unreported. More than mere law, a radical change was needed in the mindset of the society. Until the society refuses to acknowledge the reproductive rights of women and they are not treated with respect, the septic labour room would continue to have its benefactors. The forlorn corner in the labour ward would continue to suffer pain and solitude. A cursed room that stood alone in a monument of faith and healing, would keep haunting my mind with new subjects every time...

8
THE STOLEN BABY

"Live like a chameleon
Hide my colours true,
The world could not see me
And neither would you..."

A subdued dusk was casting yellow hues on the hospital as a tired sun took a quiet bow in the horizon. The hospital was probably welcoming some peace and tranquility after a day full of anxiety. Some frantic footsteps would now rest, before waking up to the hectic pace of another day. The night staff had started trickling in, taking their mandatory overs and bidding an envious goodnight to their friends as they left. Nights in the hospital were always pregnant with possibilities. However, little did anyone anticipate the drama that was soon going to unfold in the unsuspecting night.

A shrill cry broke through the silence of the quiet evening corridors. It stilled many a receding footsteps, and heads turned towards the post-natal ward. This didn't seem like the cry of a

Tripti Sharan

57

patient in pain but more of someone deeply anguished, laced with a tinge of fear. The staff on duty, along with the security people posted there, hurried towards the ward. In the second hall of the ward, a thin, dark woman was shouting frantically, 'Where is my baby? Give it back to me!' The husband was also crying, yet trying to control the hysterical woman. She wailed at him, 'You sent him to the nursery. I want my son back.' Breaking into sobs, the woman collapsed on the floor. By this time, a big crowd had gathered around the patient. People have a penchant for drama, good or bad. The woman was lifted and moved to her bed. As curious people surrounded the husband, he started narrating the incident.

He was a poor labourer and his wife had a caesarean delivery three days back. They were very happy to have a healthy baby boy. Soon after the surgery, she was shifted to the wards. They met the nurse in charge, Urmila, there. She looked after them and helped them get settled in the ward. He added that the nurse was also expecting. He didn't have any relative to help him so he had to depend on her a lot. Sometime later, the baby started crying and refused to take the mother's feed. Anxious, he called the nurse for help. She came and, after looking at the baby, told them that he needed to be kept in the nursery. She sent the husband to bring some milk powder and told him that she was shifting the baby to the nursery in the meantime. Since attendants were not allowed to enter the nursery, she asked them to enquire about the baby two days later. She assured them that they would be called, if needed. He was very grateful. She was taking care of them in spite of her advanced pregnancy state. However, today his wife was getting discharged but he had still not heard from the nursery. When he went there to find out, they were surprised and informed him that they never had his baby in the nursery. He was shocked beyond belief. He insisted that his son had been shifted there, but they refused to believe him and, rather, got irritated. The security person posted there was asked to make him leave as he was creating an unnecessary scene. Desperate, he looked for the nurse-in-charge Urmila, but was told that she had delivered and was now on maternity leave. He kept on reiterating that the nursery people had lost his newborn son.

Soon, the police was informed. The medical superintendent, the head of department, and the senior specialists too arrived. The police asked for all doctors and paramedical staff on duty on the day of the delivery, to report. It was important for the police to contact Urmila. She was called on her mobile but, initially, nobody answered. After repeated calls, she picked up the phone but sounded quiet tired. She got agitated on being asked about the patient whose baby could not be found and refused to divulge much about it, apart from accepting that she had shifted the baby to the nursery. The police insisted that she come to the police station. It was understandable that she was on a maternity leave but the police had a job to do. They didn't take kindly to her repeated attempts to thwart even a simple query. She knew she could defer no longer and was forced to comply.

By the time she reached, her case sheet had been taken out from the hospital records. It was found that Urmila was a 37-year-old, nine-months-pregnant woman and was on duty when she went into labour. She was suffering from cramps since the morning but had ignored them. It became worse, and unable to reach the labour room on time, she had to deliver in her own duty room. The doctor on duty was called in and in her notes, the doctor mentioned that Urmila appeared to be exhausted, though comfortable. She shifted her to the labour room for further examination but Urmila refused for any elaborate gynae check-ups. She was a senior nurse of the gynae department, and moreover, there were no obvious abnormalities. The doctor kept her under observation in the labour room. Later, Urmila was transferred to the post-natal ward and was discharged from there a day later.

It was past midnight when Urmila entered the police station along with her husband. She looked upset for being disturbed at this time. Many senior doctors who had known her for a long time, sympathized with her. The police took her for interrogation in a closed room. A little later what came out shocked the confidence we had in ourselves and the people we worked with. Her story rocked the very foundation of trust on which hospitals function. It showed how vulnerable we were to devious minds, especially when they happened to be one of our own people.

Urmila had confessed to her crime. A perfect plot, a foolproof plan, straight out of some thriller movie, lay exposed. She had managed to pull the wool over the eyes of the unsuspecting doctors and her colleagues, in the process, making them part of her conspiracy unknowingly. It was going to serve as a deterrent to trust anyone for a long time.

Urmila had worked in the Department of Obstetrics and Gynaecology for about ten years. She joined the hospital when she was twenty-five and, soon, won over people with her dedication and sharp clinical acumen. A year back, she had been promoted as the nurse-in-charge of the post-natal ward. However, behind this success lay a life full of struggles. She came from a poor background. Having lost her father early on, she became the sole earner of her family. After settling down her siblings, she got married and, by then, she was almost thirty. Now she had been married for seven years, but fate denied her the pleasure of motherhood. She tried everything but could not fill the void in her life. And looking after the patients and their little babies in the post-natal ward filled her with an intense longing to hold her own child in her arms. She often cribbed at the unfairness of God. The sharp barbs at home from relatives made her even more desperate.

Her growing frustration, coupled with the intense desire to have a baby, sowed seeds of a devious plot in her mind. There were lot of ignorant and illiterate people coming to the hospital and God had blessed them with an overdose of fertility. It would not harm them if she took away one of their babies! God would give them more. After all, he was the one who did not let her have her own. The thought of stealing anybody's baby did not fill her with guilt. However, she needed a master plan. She could take advantage of the overworked, and sometimes a little casual, but trusting, doctors. Her familiarity with the loopholes of the hospital was going to be her strong point.

She first needed to plan her pregnancy. She had been under the treatment of the head of the department. She decided to refrain from further medications on the pretext that she needed reprieve from the strenuous treatment cycles. The senior doctor agreed and told her to stop treatment for at least three months. A month later, she met her with the good news. Everyone was happy for her. A relaxed mind works wonders and it was not unusual for infertility patients to conceive even after stopping all treatment. She was advised some medicines and tests.

It was easy getting the blood tests and no one could be suspicious there. However, she missed the early ultrasounds, citing fears by elders at home that it would cause an abortion. Nobody could force her with that, but she needed to come for regular check-ups. A staff nurse had the privilege of seeing any doctor. Though she was registered in the unit of the head of department, she kept on shifting doctors. She needed entries in her pregnancy card, so she would register herself in the OPD (Outpatient Department) and tell the doctor that she had got her blood pressure and weight checked, and then show her reports to them. She knew that it was often difficult to feel the uterus in obese people. Most of the time, she refused to lie down and on other occasions, when the doctor was having difficulty feeling the uterus, she would get up soon, saying that she would come later when the doctor was free. It was nothing unusual with patients who were doctors or nurses. Further, hospital staffs have this habit of checking their reports themselves but not carrying them. The unsuspecting doctors didn't think much and filled her antenatal card. On the card, the pregnancy grew, uninterrupted, and officially. To avoid suspicion, she was infrequent with her check-ups and blamed her work pressure for that.

In the fifth month of pregnancy, it was time for the essential ultrasound that she could no longer avoid. She deliberately met her specialist in the corridor. The doctor was on the way to the theatre for an emergency surgery and was obviously in a hurry. Urmila stopped her, waving an ultrasound report. It was a photocopy and slightly blurred. She admitted that she had kept the original at home. The doctor could barely read it and told her to go to the clinic for check-up. Urmila smartly convinced the doctor at the clinic that she had already been seen by the senior, and she just needed to get the antenatal card filled. The overburdened doctor was rather relieved and readily complied. She could not see her name clearly on the ultrasound and Urmila once again apologized for the poor quality of the photocopy. Her familiarity with the workings of a doctor's mind managed to get her through. There was no way anyone could look through her false complains either. She had seen enough movies to make an obvious and gradually increasing swell on her body.

However, she got a little jittery and after that she didn't have any entries in the card. Whenever quizzed, she cited her busy schedule and fatigue. but assured that she had got herself checked in the labour room. The doctors and nurses were, generally, the worst patients. Moreover, the hectic pace of the hospital didn't leave much time to ponder on an unwilling patient. There was another, more willing one, waiting to be seen.

Urmila had managed to cover most milestones of her pregnancy just depending on her insight and shrewdness. Now she had to plan her delivery and this had to be her master stroke. There was no scope of any mistake, else it would easily become her waterloo. She needed to steal a newborn baby. In her supposedly last month of pregnancy, she was on a constant lookout for a vulnerable prey. There were many poor migrants who came to the hospital. Because of their illiteracy and ignorance, they lost confidence and faith in their own abilities. Moreover, they were not well-connected, either. And Urmila thrived on this weakness. On that fateful day, a poor patient, Kala Devi, entered the hospital in labour. She had no female attendant with her, only her husband. They both had migrated from their village just a month ago and had few friends. They appeared lost, unable to understand much of the formalities. Urmila had made it a point to be present in the admission room in the morning these days, on some pretext or the other. She acted as a good samaritan and helped them. Kala Devi's baby was a breech presentation and had to undergo a caesarean section. The patient was crestfallen, but Urmila was overjoyed. She couldn't have asked for more. A caesarean meant an immobilised patient, and that suited her.

By the afternoon, the patient had delivered a healthy baby boy and was shifted to the post-natal ward. Urmila tended to them lovingly, like a guardian angel. The mother was in pain and was not able to feed properly. The baby kept crying continuously. It was then that the father called for the nurse to help them. Urmila seized the chance and told him that the baby was not well and would need to be kept in the nursery. She asked him to bring some formula milk, but he didn't have much money with him. With a huge show of generosity, she offered him some cash, too. She further advised him that he should not enquire much about the baby at least for two days and instead, take care of his operated wife. Thanking his stars for meeting such a helpful lady, he left.

Urmila had already planned her next step. Those days, she was teaching the nursing students. In the morning, once Kala Devi had been shifted for surgery, she had asked her students to bring a placenta from the labour room for teaching purposes. The class was over by noon. After that, she took the baby and quietly brought him to her duty room. She gave the baby some milk and sedatives, so that he would keep sleeping, and then sent a message to her colleague that she was not feeling well. Knowing Urmila's advanced state of pregnancy, her colleague agreed to look after her ward.

At around five in the evening, she informed the labour room that she had suddenly delivered. The doctor on duty came to see her in the duty room. Urmila went to great lengths to make sure it looked like a delivery room. With precise planning and calculation, she spread some antibiotic lotion and laid the placenta near the baby. She had also made sure that she was in the right time of the month.

The doctor decided to shift her to the labour room for examination. Urmila insisted that she was perfectly normal. However, in the face of her precipitate and unaided delivery, it was imperative that she had a proper examination. After much deliberation, she agreed to be shifted. Urmila asked for her friend to get her admitted. She, in turn, sent a ward boy, and a yellow paper stamped with 'Admit in labour room' was promptly made at the admission desk.

A tired and disheveled Urmila entered the labour room in a wheelchair. Here she met another senior resident whom she knew well. The doctor congratulated Urmila and asked her to lie down. She refused, saying she had been through enough pain and didn't want to suffer any more. The doctor thought she was scared, and sympathised with her. There was no obvious sign of injury and the bleeding was not much either. Urmila promised that if she had a problem she would get the examination done. Not suspecting any foul play, the doctor agreed, but kept her under observation in the labour room. About an hour later, she was transferred to a private ward, and a day later, both the baby and his apparent mother were discharged in a healthy and stable condition amidst the good wishes of the hospital.

She had chosen her prey carefully and had planned everything meticulously. She was reveling in how easily she had managed to befool everyone. However, she had not believed that the poor couple would create a scene. Since they were poor and without contacts, she thought they would probably make a little noise but would eventually go home.

Quick action by the hospital and prompt investigation by the police nailed her, but there were many innocent bystanders who got sullied by the dirt of her deceit. The doctors who did her check-ups during her pregnancy, the ones who saw her on her presumed delivery day, the nurse, the ward boy, and the clerk who had made the papers of her admission were all suspects and co-conspirators in the eyes of law. Their role needed to be investigated. She had no qualms about destroying the lives of these people she had so selfishly used. Their careers lay jeopardised. They all tried to plead innocent, but then the law goes by facts mentioned in the case sheets. They paid the price for being trusting and casual. Even if their intent was not wrong, they now had to prove their innocence. She suffered no remorse about being a blot on a noble profession.

Later, she retracted her confession, resorting to the time-tested excuse that it was made under police pressure. The irony of our judicial system is that the truth needs to be proven 'right' in the court, and a lie, unless it's proven wrong, lingers and survives.

A pregnant night, in the hospital that had delivered more than it promised, came to an 'enlightened' end. The bemused night finally took solace in the arms of a surprised dawn. It was back to the rush hour, and busy footsteps rang through the hospital corridors once again. People jostled as they tried to reach their destination.

A staff member was seen trailing a doctor, matching her hurried steps and frantically trying to show her the reports she was carrying. The doctor signalled her to come later but finally had to stop. She could be seen leafing through the staff member's reports. Well, some things just never change!

9
THE STRANGER

"Your passion holds the stormy flights,
You are there even when I sleep all night.
The world doesn't know and cannot see,
But stranger, I know you follow me ..."
(From my poem *The Stranger*, published in the book *Spectrum*)

The radio was playing a hit number. The sweet voice of the singer filled the air as she crooned softly. Yet, it failed to soothe me, and I stared at the hospital corridors nervously. Dusk had settled in and was casting mysterious shadows. I shrugged, and walked slowly. A pricking sensation on my neck forced me to stop and look back. Except for a few attendants sitting and chatting with each other, there was no stranger lurking in the dark, ready to spring at me. The incidences of the past few days were making my imagination work overtime.

A patient had been brought from a nearby village in a critical condition. She was suffering from eclampsia, an undesirable but largely preventable complication of high blood pressure during pregnancy. It was quite prevalent in anaemic patients and those who did not have proper check-ups during pregnancy. Despite the best efforts, neither the baby nor the patient could be saved. Her husband refused to accept this. He lost his mental balance, sprung out a knife, and ran after the duty doctors. They were all women. The hospital took pride in its ancient heritage, which meant that there were hardly any proper bolts or locks. Most of the doors could not withstand even a friendly kick. Fortunately, the ward *bai* alerted the doctors and they ran off towards the recovery room outside the operation theatre which was the only room that boasted of some secure doors and windows. The husband, mad with grief, lunged after them, flashing his knife dangerously. Till then the security and other staff had been informed. They all rushed towards the room. The man was overpowered, but not before the doctors inside spent some tense and anxious moments, fearing for their lives.

Sometimes, revelling in our profession, we forget we are still the physically weaker sex. This incident had laid bare the non-existent security for doctors and the callous attitude of some people towards the medical fraternity. It also showed how vulnerable our profession made us in the hands of disgruntled people. Every patient walking into a hospital hopes to survive. But every time a patient dies, it cannot be the fault of the doctors. However, there are very few who are willing to accept this. These days, our profession makes news for all the wrong reasons. This incident flared up the tension between the doctors and the administration. There were a lot of protests and eventually the security was beefed up, but not before the doctors threatened to go on strike. Now a police post kept a vigil just outside the labour room. Armed guards were also deployed. Hopefully, they were here to stay.

Fortunately, I didn't get much time to ponder. I had reached the triage. An interesting patient awaited me. A tribal woman in the last month of pregnancy had been pierced by an arrow in her village. The villagers suspected that she was under the influence of bad spirits. Probably, they were witch hunting. It was rampant in some villages. She had travelled for two days in a bus, without lying down, to reach our hospital. The baby had died and we strongly suspected a ruptured uterus. She was, understandably, exhausted. Yet, there was no fear in her eyes.

A herculean task lay ahead to save the brave woman. It was a challenge giving her anaesthesia as she could not even lie down. Some gruelling hours later the arrow was removed, along with the dead baby, uterus and a part of her gut. The surgery was successful but exhausting. However, there can never be a bigger high than saving a life. In those moments, fighting against all odds, we are united with the ultimate divine force that drives our lives. We call him The Almighty. And in that moment, everything else was forgotten, our joys as well as our fears, our smiles as well as our tears!

The woman intrigued me. I wanted to know more about her but she was still groggy under the effects of anaesthesia and I didn't want to intrude upon her privacy.

I was just about to get out of the operation theatre when my mobile beeped. There was a message from an unsaved number.

'You have destroyed me!'

Who was this? What was I supposed to have done? A chill ran down my spine. Was I being stalked? I looked around. I couldn't see anyone. There were so many ghost calls these days in the labour room. There was a string of obscenities but, strangely, only when picked up by a female doctor. Last night, a crude voice, almost in an illiterate tone, had used medical terms pertaining to female anatomy with so much vulgarity that I shuddered. Someone inside the hospital was a pervert. The incident was reported to the administration and they had promised action.

Those days, the story of Aruna Shanbaug was much in news. I shivered. I didn't want to think of her at this time. The presence of armed guards in the wards was reassuring. I had a call from the post-operative ward and, after that, I planned to go to the nursery for some research work. After finishing my rounds, I headed straight for the nursery. I took the register to the doctor's room where I could work uninterrupted. I was just closing the register when a ward boy entered. I had seen him earlier too, hovering in the wards. Something about him made me uncomfortable. Maybe it was the way he was looking at me, obliquely, or the way he walked, covering one side of his face with his hands. He looked dirty and a little sick. I didn't like him, but standing in front of him in a narrow duty room, I had no choice. Suddenly, the room filled with a disturbing aura. Instinctively, I knew I had to get out. But he was blocking my way. I got out of my chair and, crossing him carefully, came to stand at the door.

I asked him in an authoritative tone, '*Kya kaam hai?*' ('What do you want?')

He didn't say anything; just looked at me in a creepy way. A strange fear gripped me but I didn't let it show. He slowly took out a piece of crumpled paper from the pocket of his trousers. Not understanding much of what was happening, I opened the paper. In a dirty handwriting, but legibly enough, was splayed one word – '*Nirodh*'. I cringed. He could have easily asked the nurses of the post-natal ward for it. For a fleeting moment, it crossed my mind that he might actually be needing them, but I pushed the thought away. My intuitions were ringing warning bells. How dare he creep over me like this at this time!

The nervous apprehensions of the past few days and the haunting fear all came together with a force, flaring up an anger so intense that I raised my hand and hit him on his back. Needing a physical outlet for the sheer disgust I was feeling, I kept on punching him. He shielded himself even as he grovelled. Hitting him, I hurt myself, too, but nothing could stop me.

I dragged him to the post-natal ward where a senior nurse was sitting. The nurse scolded him but the pathetic creature kept on covering his eyes and tilting his face. Bereft of all energy, I didn't know what to do with him. Strangely, he looked as if he was relishing every blow and that enraged me further. I left

him with the ward nurse and called up my friends. They rushed
to the ward. I was almost in tears, but still managed to quickly
brief them. They took him away. Instead of fear, there was still
a sick gaze in his eyes as he looked at me. Unable to face him,
I turned back and went to my ward. He was roughened up in
the boy's hostel thoroughly before being reported to the medical
superintendent. He promised action and transferred him to the
male wards, which was in a different building and away from
our hospital. I was relieved, though still uneasy with him being
around. I wanted a more severe punishment but, according to the
authorities, his crime was not very big. There were strong unions
and the administration was wary of messing with them. A strange
hesitation and an illogical shame prevented me from charging
him with perversion and implicating him as the person behind
the vulgar calls made to the labour room. My friends chided me
for being a namby-pamby. They reassured me that he would
never come near me again and I tried my best to get convinced.
The days that followed showed no trace of him and, slowly, I let
go of my fears. The phantom calls to the labour room had also
stopped. The messages gradually retreated to a forgotten corner
of my mind and life, once again, moved to the routine track.

I had just entered home when my phone buzzed. I fumbled
within my purse and looked at the unknown number. Flinging off
my purse, I answered the call but then froze! 'You have spoiled
my life,' a stranger accused me bitterly.

I whispered back, 'Who are you?'

He continued, 'Why did you do this to me?'

This was getting weird. I could make no sense of what was
going on. At any other time, I wouldn't have continued the call,
but now I was overcome with panic.

'What have I done?' With a sense of forbidding, I held my
breath.

'There is no peace in my family. You have falsely implicated
me.' His accusation stung without any reason.

'I don't even know you; have never met you,' I replied, uneasily. Was it a madman on loose? My better senses again warned me to cut-off the call.

'You saw my niece, Zarine, a few months back.'

'So what if I did? I didn't do anything wrong!'

Where was all this leading to? I was getting even more confused. A small girl, who had come with her mother and aunt, entered my mind.

'You accused me of molesting her!'

'How can I do that? I didn't even know she had an uncle.'

'Then why did you say such things?'

I was zapped and tried hard to recollect.

Zarine was a small girl, about eight years old. Her mother was worried'that Zarine kept having irritation in, and discharge from, her private parts. She was quite concerned about her. I had a quick look and everything looked all right. I reassured her mother, but then she started telling me about the news of girls being abused. On an impulse, I asked her to be a little careful with people she goes out with. These were bad times we lived in and she was still so young. Her mother told me about her school van driver but he had been with them for a long time and was a trusted person. They had checked with her teachers and school friends, too. I advised her to be careful with people she was in touch with at home, also. One could not trust anyone these days. Her mother agreed wholeheartedly and promised to be careful. With that, they left and it was all forgotten. I never thought that I would have to bear the fall out of a simple and rational discussion. Was I to suffer the side effects of my own advice?

'My family is destroyed! You have broken the trust! My own niece! How could you, doctor?'

My fear had now given place to anger and irritation. It was time to be a bit firm.

'Look mister, whosoever you are, I gave a purely professional advice. There was nothing personal about it. I still don't know anything about the family of Zarine. I simply asked her mother to be careful with the people her daughter is in contact with, because we keep seeing children getting assaulted by people known to them. I never implied that she had been assaulted by you. If her mother doubts you, chooses not to trust you, it's not my doing! You should be questioning your sister-in-law rather than sending me anonymous messages. They are unwarranted and an intrusion of my privacy. I can report you for that. It was never my intention to hurt you or break your family. Please do not condemn me for a crime I never committed. Maybe it's time you sat down with your family and sorted out your problems in private.'

I never heard his response for the phone went quiet. Later, I was berated by my friends for overreacting. The whole episode kept haunting me even though I tried to make light of it. I prayed the message had hit home. A faceless man had intruded into my comfort zone and had somehow broken my peace. As doctors, we are so used to giving our opinions, sometimes too assertively. Maybe it was time I learned to mind my own business and refrain from unnecessarily poking my head everywhere.

A month passed by and, thankfully, there were no messages. One day while on rounds, my mobile beeped again. 'I am a condemned man today. It's all because of you!'

I was both shocked and angry. Frankly, I didn't know who I was dealing with. Maybe, he was a sick person after all. Maybe he wanted to shift all the blame on me and be free himself. He had declared me the culprit and refused to listen to logic. Who knows? His sister-in-law might be having genuine reasons to doubt him!

Once again, I was advised to report him to the police. I didn't want any kind of interaction with an irrational man. I simply blocked his number. Though he knew where I worked, I prayed that he would keep his distance and not trouble me further. In any case, the option of going to the police was always open. I kicked myself for sweating over a man who was either sick, or just having fun at my expense. Ignoring is an art and a saving grace in a majority of situations, and I should have made use of it. After all, I had better things to do in my life!

I focused my attention on the woman sitting in front of me. Oh, the same tribal woman! She had come back for her post-operative check-up. She was definitely looking much better, and once again I was impressed by her captivating smile.

'So, how are you doing? Back to your village?' I couldn't help smiling back at her.

'I am fine, ma'am. Where else will I go? All my life I have lived there.'

'Aren't you scared of living there now?'

She laughed suddenly. 'Why, crimes don't happen here, ma'am? Your city makes more news than mine.'

I just looked at her. She had hit home.

'For how long can you run? And who all do you run from?' she continued.

'How did it all happen?'

'I was trying hard to conceive. My sister told me to get a "ritual" done to appease the Gods for that. Soon thereafter, I conceived. However, I was in my last month of pregnancy when my neighbour's wife, who was pregnant, went into labour and delivered a stillborn girl child. Around the same time, my sister, who was also pregnant, delivered a premature, deformed baby. Doctors said it was anencephaly (when a baby is born without parts of the brain and skull), but the villagers thought it was a demon. Soon, it was presumed all over the village that we were witches and performed black magic. We were blamed for everything that went wrong in our village.'

I listened to her.

'They might harm you again. You should really leave the village.'

'And let them win? I will stay back and fight, even if I die.'

I admired her grit and courage. She had travelled miles in such a vulnerable condition, overcoming fear; a difficult terrain; and friends who had turned foes, victims to their own ignorance and superstition. And here I was, seeing shadows in the dark, troubled by voices from far!

That day, I, an empowered woman living in privileged surroundings, took lessons from a simple, illiterate woman coming from an underprivileged village. Maybe I drew strength from her, but what rose that day was the spirit of a woman; a force that can be dented, but can never be broken; a power – the essence of a woman – that has survived and built civilizations.

A woman, defying all odds, smiled victorious once again!

10
THE DELHI GIRL

"Let me feel once again,
Let me heal once again,
Let me break the chains,
They only bring more pain.
Do not clip my wings,
Let me ride with the winds..."

'Madam, she is so sick. I don't know what's wrong with her.'

The anxiety from the other end of the phone was almost palpable. The voice sounded urgent and familiar. I was getting immune to the presumption by most patients that we can recognize over the telephone, not only them, but even their husbands.

'Who is this?' I asked patiently.

He was immediately apologetic. 'I am Rajbir. Gurneeta's husband. You delivered our baby about two years back.'

Living in Delhi, I had realized the fascination the city holds for such names. A slight change in letters and you have Gurmeet, Gurmeeta, Gurneet, Gurpreet, Gurpreeta and many more interesting possibilities. Delhi loves to dabble with them, and later confuse the already overworked brain of a doctor!

'What happened to her?'

'She is not speaking... can't even get up. There is a sudden bout of weakness. I really don't know what is wrong with her.' He sounded perplexed. I could well imagine a whole lot of things and advised him to bring her to the hospital.

An hour later, a downcast Gurneeta was ushered in by her much worried husband into my clinic. I tried to recognize her. Yeah, she looked familiar. However, I recalled a much different, feisty girl. She had breezed into my clinic about five years back. A bubbly girl, she loved to throw caution to the winds. However, now stripped of all vitality, I stared at a very different person. She refused to meet my eyes, as if she was ashamed of something. Over the years, I had seen so many emotions crossing her face, but never anything like this. Something was terribly amiss.

'Hello, Gurneeta.' I tried to talk to her but she could barely whimper. She raised her eyes at me and then looked away. Women were prone to mood swings and psychiatric disorders during pregnancy.

'There is no possibility of a pregnancy,' her husband told me, hesitantly. He looked sadly at my questioning eyes but didn't elaborate further.

She was twenty-six years old, with a two year-old-son at home. A sudden bout of weakness yesterday and she refused to get up. She could barely talk. They took her to a nearby nursing home. She was put on some intravenous fluids but she didn't improve. I could not find physical evidence of any disease.

'Could she be stressed out?'

Her husband denied any disagreement in the family.

'She was much quieter the past few days. Things were not the same between us any more. I attributed it to the demands of parenthood that was keeping us away. Our son was not letting her rest properly, or sleep either. My own work made things worse, but my mother was always with her,' he admitted reluctantly.

Maybe it was rubbing on his conscience. They were always such a close-knit family.

But motherhood was no easy cake. I decided to refer her to a physician. They readily agreed.

All the while, there was hardly any word from the once-so-lively patient.

I was forced to ask, 'Aren't you happy, Gurneeta?'

'I feel so weak,' was all she could whisper, as if the mere effort was hurting her. I was baffled.

They went to see the physician, promising to be back with his report. As I waited for them, I couldn't help going back to the first time I had met her, nearly five years ago…

My last appointment was scheduled at 5 pm. It was 5.30 pm now and she was still nowhere to be seen. I was about to leave my room when the door was pushed open and a pretty girl walked in, dropping a cheerful greeting. I raised my eyebrows and she said apologetically, 'Ma'am! I am Gurneeta. I was supposed to be here at 5 pm, but you know Delhi's bad traffic.'

'I know. It's such a convenient thing,' I replied sarcastically. She grinned. Her smile was actually infectious and I couldn't help smiling back.

'Madam, I am about twenty years old and soon going into a relationship. I wanted some contraceptive advice.'

I was impressed. This one had come at the right time. 'Are you going to marry?' I asked before I could stop myself.

'I am not very sure,' she laughed and replied candidly. I was seeing many young girls these days and had started admiring the gutsy Delhi girls. There was a scarcity of proper sex education and parents were still reluctant to talk about it. The changing values in our society were putting these girls into real danger. AIDS, the only sexually-transmitted infection the majority of them knew, was just the tip of the iceberg. A pregnancy at this age was equally traumatic. It was not my job to judge them or teach them morality but give a sound medical advice.

Sometime back, a young girl was brought in the casualty. She had been out with friends to a party, later got queasy, and didn't remember much. Probably drinks and drugs! She was loaded with guilt and was almost hysterical, surrounded by a teary mother and an emotionally-wounded father. It was a tough task controlling all of them. At times, I pitied these young people. They were caught in a crossfire between traditional parents, daring peers, and an enticing social media that lured them. At least this girl had the good sense to come and talk to a doctor. It was much better than pouring one's heart out on the internet, and filling oneself with a half-baked truth. We had a long discussion where I explained a lot many things. She, too, was open on her part. I warned her that she shouldn't come here with a pregnancy. She grinned again and left. It was her spirit and infectious smile that lingered in my mind for long.

The hot summers were back with a ferocity and it was a bliss to stay indoors in a centrally-cooled hospital with no fear of power cuts. The summer vacations, plus the hot winds, had actually reduced the number of patients in the outdoor clinics, especially in the afternoons. I was ready to leave, when I heard someone calling me. I turned around and was pleasantly surprised to see Gurneeta standing there. Was it a tinge of nervousness that marred her beautiful eyes? I sat expectantly, waiting for her to speak. You don't pay a courtesy visit to the doctor.

'I am pregnant!' she blurted out.

I stared at her. 'You didn't listen to me at all,' I said accusingly.

'I was scared of taking the regular contraceptive pills. It would have made my parents suspicious. My boyfriend told me that I could take another kind of pill,' she hesitated a little before she told me the name. I disliked that immensely. I had told her that it was an emergency pill to be used in extreme situations only.

'It was an emergency.' She was defiant.

'Really?'

Well, emergency to a patient is entirely different from emergency to a doctor.

'We discussed other options, too.'

I replied angrily. She fumbled and her voice trailed off. I understood, and wanted to swear rudely. An emergency contraceptive pill was such a convenient excuse to cover up irresponsible behaviour. A rampantly misused drug; its over-the-counter availability was a sign of our country's frustration over a rising population.

Overriding our disappointments, we sat down to think of a way out. She wanted an abortion. I wanted some attendant, preferably a family member, who she could take into confidence. I was against doing something undercover. If things went wrong, I would very easily be labelled as the money-grabbing doctor. So, I wrote down some tests and advised her to come the next day with some relative.

The following day I saw her waiting for me. No traffic woes today! However, there was no relative with her. A lanky youth suddenly appeared beside her.

'I am her senior in the office,' he said, a little too boldly. Looking at my raised eyebrows, he hastily added, 'I am twenty-three years old.' Needless to say, I was impressed by his age.

She refused to inform her family. She was an adult and, legally, could have an abortion anywhere. Besides, I didn't want to push her to some unqualified person. So, we sat down and I explained to them the procedure and possible complications. She didn't have much choice, yet I appreciated her boldness in accepting everything calmly, rather than give in to histrionics. She could not have her medicines at home and I didn't want her to be at any random fast food joint, writhing in pain.

'It is much practical and safer to be in the hospital. But this is a private hospital and like the majority of things in life, this doesn't come free, either.'

'That's fine ma'am. The boyfriend will pay,' she brightly informed me. I couldn't help smiling at the implied justice. At least, she had kept her sense of humour intact.

They stayed in the hospital for a day and were the cynosure of all eyes. Our young female residents gushed over her cute friend who kept holding her hands. They were ready to bet that the boyfriend was past and this guy would fill in soon. On my part, I accepted that I couldn't comprehend present day relationships. In the evening, she went home to parents who remained oblivious to her day-long pain and trauma, and ignorant of something as important as pregnancy in their daughter's life.

It was more than a year later that I saw her again. This time, a visibly happy, newly-married Gurneeta waited for me. I refrained from asking if he was the boyfriend, the friend who held her hand, or neither!

'I have been married for about six months now and want to get pregnant. My husband is the eldest son and there are lots of family pressures.'

For the first time she talked about her parents. 'I had a wonderful marriage. My parents spent generously and gave me a big dowry.'

I looked at her questioningly. She laughed uneasily. 'This earns me respect in the eyes of my husband and his family. Moreover, in a way, it is my share in my parents' property, isn't it?'

I raised an eyebrow. She flushed, but kept quiet. I wondered who was teaching her these things. Her mother-in-law hovered around and hardly left her alone. I failed to comprehend the obsession people had for having grandchildren. Her husband, a new guy I had not met earlier, entered the chamber discreetly and hardly spoke, probably not being used to speaking in front of his mother. I missed the chirpy, *bindaas* (carefree) girl I once knew, but in all fairness, I couldn't say that she was unhappy. She had probably adjusted to her circumstances, which was not a bad thing to do after all. I reassured them that they just needed to be a little patient. They left, happy and satisfied. Back to the mundane routine of my profession, I was lost in the challenges God keeps throwing our way. I forgot Gurneeta.

But then, like a wisp of fresh air, she walked into my clinic a year later. She was about two months pregnant and accompanied by a beaming mother-in-law and husband. I was happy for her. Later, she was quite regular with her check-ups. Though her husband always appeared scarce in the presence of his dominating mother, I could see that he cared for her. Gurneeta looked radiant. She was enthusiastic about every minute thing, like recording the baby's first heartbeat they heard, to saving the ultrasound pictures. We encouraged couples to come together for the check-ups. It helped them bond better and grow as a family. But here, it was difficult to get past her omnipresent mother-in-law. I hoped their relationship was strong enough to withstand this constant intrusion.

Soon, Gurneeta was into her seventh month of pregnancy and we were moving towards the end of the year. Somehow, the baby had stopped gaining weight.

'Are you taking good diet and rest?' I asked.

'There is hardly any time to take rest at home,' she confessed. She sounded a bit jittery.

'Ma'am, may I know the sex of the baby?' she suddenly asked. 'I desperately wish it to be a girl, even if it makes others unhappy,' she said quietly. I was startled. She continued, 'If I have a boy, it will strain my father. He will have to give expensive gifts once again. He has two more daughters to look after and he has to bear the cost of this delivery, too. Every time he is forced to do something like this, a part of me dies and I lose respect for myself.'

I could understand her stress now.

'Girls are a liability in my culture. Even the funeral has to be arranged by the father. Inspite of earning well, I can't help my parents as the mere thought is repugnant to my family.' She couldn't stop the bitterness from creeping into her voice. I felt sad for her but I couldn't interfere in her family matters. I wished that she had been more assertive, and stopped things in the beginning itself. Sadly, the husband remained a mute spectator in a majority of Indian households. His larger than life role as a son marred the growth of a husband.

There were no further outbursts on her subsequent visits. Maybe she had resigned to her fate, or maybe things had improved at home. In the hospital, they were always a picture of solidarity with no hint of any discord. It could well be my imagination but, at times, I saw a forced smile and wariness on her tired face. Her laughs were now few and forced. Pregnancy is a strange physiology in a woman's life. It sometimes clams you up and makes you moody as hell.

A few days before her delivery date, Gurneeta went into labour. She tolerated her pains well. We encouraged husbands to be a part of the delivery process and support their wives, but her mother-in-law didn't allow him to enter the labour room. She was adamant that her son was not capable of withstanding all this stress. The couple remained silent in mute acceptance of her domination.

Oblivious to the turmoil outside, life opened its baby eyes with a loud cry. Gurneeta had delivered a baby boy, much to the joy of everyone. Desire for a male child is global but India beats the world in being the craziest. Gurneeta was also happy, enjoying the moment of prestige that being the mother of a male child, momentarily bestowed upon her. The whole family fussed over her. We discharged a healthy baby and a happy mother a few days later.

On her next visit, I could make out the telltale signs of sleepless nights.

'You have so many helping hands at home.'

'I have to fend for myself all alone. My husband sleeps in another room as instructed by his mother. He has to go for work next day,' she informed me, dispelling my notions. She bore no grudges. It wasn't for me to judge, but I wished he was around when she needed him the most. Post-partum (post-delivery) depression was common in women and they buckled under the demands of motherhood, all too often. However, once again, the doctor had to mind her own business and keep quiet.

A month later, Gurneeta came to see me again. She had come from her parents' home this time. She was doing well medically, but she was upset about something and wanted to vent. 'It pains me when I strain my father financially but things are beyond my control now and I have been succumbing to the pressures for long. My husband is a nice person but is too meek to protest, or maybe he secretly likes the lavish gifts he receives. Even my parents agree that this was a duty the society had imposed on them,' she reluctantly admitted.

I grimly told her, 'You have a son now. The least you can do is to not follow such customs when you get him married.'

She laughed hard, and, just for a while, I caught a glimpse of the old Gurneeta. 'If I live that long!' she sobered up. That was the last time I had seen her...

My brief mental sojourn was broken by the sound of a wheelchair. Gurneeta had come back. I called up the physician. He confirmed my suspicion of this being a psychological breakdown. They needed psychiatric consultation. Her husband looked broken as I explained to him. 'I hope you understand that this is no low blood pressure or any viral illness. It has been simply brought about by years of neglect.' He opened his mouth to protest but kept quiet. The fear of losing his wife had probably made him wiser. He said quietly, 'I might not have been a good husband but I do care for her a lot.' I believed the sincerity in his voice. Simple words were more convincing than loud declarations of love. Both of them needed to grow out of their respective limitations. He from his mother's shadows, and she from her present state. Considering the stigma of mental illness, the most important component was acceptance of the disease. At least, there he had not lagged behind. Life had taught him a lesson and I was sure he would not fail this time.

However, Gurneeta was a different proposition. The look of sheer helplessness in her eyes tore at my heart. In the years that I had known her, from 'I don't give a damn!', to her sheepish looks when she had an abortion all on her own, and, later, to her calm acceptance as a submissive wife in her husband's family, she had lived it all. I had witnessed her transformation. But one day, her resilience broke, and the dam burst! If only we realize that freedom and modernity was not only about looks, dresses, and relationships, but the thoughts and essence that we carry as assertive and self-respecting women.

Soon, they left. The crunching sound of the receding wheelchair strangely comforted my troubled thoughts. Maybe it was reassuring me that it would bring back the lively girl I so admired once upon a time. Probably this time, 'the Delhi girl' would stay forever…

11
SHE OPENED HER EYES

"A plethora of stories untold,
A myriad of emotions unfold;
But unaware she slept
Until she opened our eyes…"

The shrill voice of the telephone disturbed the calm efficiency of the clinic till I couldn't ignore it any longer. 'Ma'am, *ICU staff bol rahi hai* (ICU staff speaking),' I smiled at the thick Malayali accent. We had plenty of nurses from Kerala and their scarce knowledge of Hindi both amused and exasperated us. 'Madam, a young girl has been referred from another hospital. She is on a ventilator.' The distress in the voice from the other side was obvious, but what could a gynaecologist do there? It was not a very usual thing for my speciality, as we generally didn't deal with critical patients. Our patients were young and healthy and, barring cancers which, fortunately, were being seen by the oncology department now, there were very less complications these days.

'Is she pregnant?'

'No, ma'am,' replied the nurse.

I grumbled, not really wanting to go to the ICU. But a call from ICU could not be ignored and I had no choice.

As always I was gripped by a sense of awe when I entered the ICU. It is this place where life turns really bare, stripped off all the masks. Our emotions were our true cosmetics. Illness, fear, pain, and grief left us undisguised, and had a universal expression. I could see the same expression on all the patients and their attendants. One day, we all have to go. But are we bold enough to accept that? As doctors, we could still not avert the inevitable, but advanced technology and better medical knowledge had allowed us to keep it hanging a bit. Ultimately, we, too, were a check post in the hands of the Smart Guy living above who made us do his little tricks.

I was hurried in by a tired looking resident. The chief intensivist and his whole team were surrounding the patient. On close quarters, I could make out a young girl on a ventilator. The tubes, masks, and the intravenous fluid sets hid her face as she lay unconscious with her eyes closed. The chief intensivist gave me a welcome smile and quickly briefed me. 'Hello dear, we are sorry to drag you into this, but we are in a fix. This girl was brought here in a critical condition. When she came, her pulse and blood pressure were unrecordable. We are maintaining her vitals with difficulty.'

'Why is she here?' I interrupted.

He smiled sarcastically. 'We don't know. All I know is that she studies in Delhi and lives in a hostel. She was with her boyfriend till last night. After dinner, she started feeling sick and giddy. He rushed her to the hospital. But by the time they reached, she was in a state of shock, with no pulse or blood pressure recordable. She had to be put on a ventilator. We are not sure if it's a homicide or a suicide. A toxic screen was sent but that, too, has come negative. We have also informed the police, to rule out any foul play.'

'Well, what do you want from me?' I asked.

'Just to make sure there is no problem from your side that could have caused this,' he replied coolly. Now that was so typical.

It just has to be a woman, and everyone starts suspecting it to be a gynaecological cause. Yet, an ectopic pregnancy (a pregnancy outside the uterus) causing massive haemorrhage and shock could be a possibility. But was there indeed a pregnancy? Even as I asked myself this, I realized the futility of my question. The one who knew the truth lay in a deep sleep. Seeking some desperate answers, I asked for the boyfriend to be called in.

Not wanting to waste my time, I decided to get on with my examination. I could see the young woman bound by tubes, holding on to her life. She was thinly built. Her abdomen was strangely tense and bloated. Was it blood, or just fluid collected due to organ failure? I was worried. However, as I touched her, I was shocked by what I could feel. I could bet my life that what I felt was a small fetal (baby's) head. And as I absorbed this piece of information, it also sunk in that this was a nearly seven-month-pregnancy that lay almost unidentified and the patient lay in shock for no apparent cause. The only person now, who could provide us a clue, was the one who claimed to be her boyfriend.

The ICU staff ushered in a nervous guy who looked not more than twenty-five years old. By now he had probably become used to telling his story. Sounding a little bored, he repeated almost the same one as told by our intensivist. However, my ears picked up that the fact that she was suffering from headache, and had also vomited, before they rushed to the hospital. I wondered if he had poisoned her or injured her, but I brushed off the nagging thought.

They had known each other for two years and kept meeting off and on. He lived in Punjab and helped his father run his business there. The girl belonged to a different state and lived alone in Delhi. They stayed in hotels whenever they met.

I looked up at him – a short, thin, jittery guy who called himself Sameer.

'This is a private hospital. Would you be able to afford this?'

He suddenly sounded very confident. 'Don't worry! She is from a very rich family.'

I looked at him suspiciously. He shifted uneasily. 'I have informed her sister.'

'Your father?' I prodded. He lowered his eyes.

'Do you realise you could be in trouble if she doesn't survive?' I could see he was scared but he kept quiet. I moved on to things which were more relevant to me. I asked him if she had ever been pregnant. He hesitated, then replied, 'Yes, once. But she underwent abortion.' And that was three months back.

'Well, she happens to be pregnant now!'

It was as if I had dropped a bomb. Suddenly, he appeared to be at a loss. 'Pregnant! She can't be!' he squealed. 'I have not met her for the last three months. I can't be the father.' It was the wrong thing to say even if it relieved him from the present impasse. And I guess he realised that the moment he said it and saw irritation cross my face. Typical of men! The woman was lying unconscious and the one she was having an affair with denied being the father.

'That's not important to us. Since you are the only one with her, we have to inform you. And it is not for us to explain that, in any case. The one who can do that is unconscious,' I added rudely. However, I wanted to know more about the pregnancy.

He went on. 'She was just about three months overdue and had gone to see a doctor for abortion. I don't know the name and couldn't be there physically but I paid her about eight thousand rupees,' he claimed proudly, as if that absolved him of his guilt.

'Are you sure she underwent that abortion?' I asked him.

'She was given some medicines and she bled for a few days, so she must have had it.' He sounded quite confidant of that. I looked at him doubtfully. Either the girl was lying or she had been duped by someone. Or, who knows, maybe this guy was the guilty one.

'Well, she was about seven months pregnant and, by all accounts, this appears to be the continuation of the same pregnancy.'

I had to inform him that and left him at it, letting him come to his own conclusions. There were doubts crossing his face. Feeling a twinge of sympathy for him, I turned to our radiologist who had just arrived. He confirmed a 28-weeks-live pregnancy, but we still didn't know what was wrong with the mother.

Soon, the blood and urine test reports came in. There were large amounts of albumin in the urine. This meant that the patient was probably in this condition because of high blood pressure during pregnancy. The dilemma, now, was how to prove conclusively that she ever had high blood pressure when it had never been recorded. Moreover, she had reported to our hospital with an unrecordable blood pressure. It is well known that this can go undetected and lead to complications with those who do not have proper check-ups during pregnancy. What we were seeing could be the end result of that condition.

In the absence of any other positive results and no record of any pre-existing medical illness or, rather, no relative to give a history, the presumptive diagnosis was pregnancy-induced high blood pressure, complicated by eclampsia (which meant convulsions and probable brain oedema). Now, this demanded immediate delivery by surgery, else this young girl would die. Doing surgery on such a critically ill patient always ran with the risk of 'death on table'. An informed consent for DOT, as we called it, had to be taken. A young, unmarried girl with no friends or parents but a reluctant boyfriend, who would run at the first hint, was a very tricky situation. If anything went wrong, all hell would break loose and we would easily be declared the villains of the story.

However, this was a young life, and had to be saved. Not left with much support, we decided to go by our own instincts. The customary explaining of informed risks to her unwilling attendant felt like banging our own heads. We informed our medical superintendent and, along with two other doctors, signed the consent on behalf of missing attendants. It was quite something, taking the signature of the boyfriend who behaved as if he should have been anywhere but there.

It was getting late. I had to inform my family, too. They never liked my long spells of absence, but my kids had learned to use it to the best of their advantage, which meant extra hours playing on the computer or watching television.

We remembered, just in the nick of time, to inform the paediatrician as well. One could not even guarantee him a live baby, but then, it was important for him to be there. So, in the spirit of our noble profession, he also said goodbye to his busy clinic and joined us in the operation theatre.

The patient was already on a ventilator so not much time was wasted in anaesthesia. In the theatre, the most tense person is usually the anaesthetist. His career depends not only on his own expertise, but on the expertise of the surgeon and the condition of the patient.

To my dismay, when we were on the verge of giving that first nick, the anaesthetist shouted, 'Hey, wait! Her oxygen pressure is dropping.'

My hands stilled. I had never operated on a dead patient. Something inside me revolted. The origin of the caesarean section lay in an old custom of the ancient Romans, called *lex caesarica* (Caesar's law), where you don't bury the mother and baby together, and so, one does a caesarean on the dead mother and takes out the baby. There were some cases reported of the mother dying and the baby being taken out in a desperate bid to save it. I had never been in such a dramatic situation, and withdrew. I couldn't do it. But then how would we explain if she died without delivering? It would seem that we did nothing to save her. Listening to an inner voice, and with a nod from the anaesthetist, we decided to go ahead. I said a silent prayer and went on. She was completely white, and it was as if we were indeed operating on the dead.

Within minutes, we had the baby out. To our surprise, we took out a preterm, but healthy, crying baby girl. And like a miracle, as we went on with the closing, her oxygen pressure started improving. By the time we shifted her to ICU, we were optimistic. It was past midnight but it was as if we had won a battle. Completely drained, but happy at the way things had turned out, it was time to retire.

The baby was looked after by the nurses, in the nursery. She was preterm and needed a lot of care. Her boyfriend was hardly around on the excuse that there was not much he could do.

The next few days saw her getting better, but her attendants remained scarce. As claimed by the boyfriend, her rich relatives never turned up. A younger sister came, but soon left on the pretext of her exams. A friend from the hostel used to visit her often. All of us at the hospital were very sympathetic of the helpless and wronged girl. On the pretext of some important work, her boyfriend left, promising to be back soon. Just before he was leaving, he offered generously, 'I will take some time to come back. From my side, you are free to give up the baby for adoption.'

We smarted under his irresponsible attitude and ignorance of the law of the land. In his haste to get rid of the baby, he had forgotten that it was a punishable offence to abandon your child.

Meanwhile, the girl steadily improved and was soon out of the ICU. We were surprised to know that her boyfriend had given us a false name. And all those who thought she was a woman 'wronged', were in for a shock. She refused to even acknowledge the pregnancy. She accepted her relationship with her boyfriend, but there was something strange in her behaviour whenever we talked about the baby. She didn't want to have anything to do with it and would turn away, the moment we mentioned it. She kept a stoic silence and refused to utter a word. From a helpless woman who lay with her eyes closed, she turned into a cold woman who refused to open her eyes to the reality. She outrightly rejected her baby.

The hospital grudgingly had to accept that no one was going to turn up to pay the bills. Once again in the name of our noble profession, we had to lay aside the tense gruelling moments spent with her. There is no price to save lives and, sadly, neither is there a price to be paid to stay away from your family. I marvelled at the demands the society makes on our profession, in the name of nobility. A couple can afford to have an affair, spend time in hotels, spend money on quacks, but when it comes to the doctors, they didn't have any money or any family in the world. If things had gone wrong, we would have easily become the money-grabbing greedy doctors. But then, apart from carrying the legacy of our noble profession, there was not much a poor doctor could do.

Our staff was often advising her to get married to her boyfriend, but she simply ruled out the option. She didn't hold him responsible for any wrong, either. Her calm acceptance of the situation was baffling. I tried to explain to her the implication of her condition, especially for her future life and subsequent pregnancies, but to no avail. Despite repeatedly asking about the so-called doctor she had gone to for her abortion, she maintained a rigid silence. I had my own prototypes of an aggrieved woman and she didn't quite fit into either. She asked to be discharged, but we couldn't let her go as there was no one to take care of her and she had been so critically ill. She, on her part, thought the hospital was keeping her back against her will as she had not paid the bills. Every time we went to see her, she would say, 'I have a gold chain. Take that. Or you can take my kidneys.' She had no idea how much saving her had cost us. Anyway, not expecting the woman that she was fast becoming, to understand, we just requested her for one thing.

'There is someone you owe, here. Go and see your baby. She has done nothing wrong. Let her feel that she is loved and wanted. Just visit her once. She is an adorable baby.'

However, I realized that I was just talking to her rude back, as always.

I failed to understand her. Maybe she didn't want to accept what she had done. She might be in some kind of denial, or else she might be thinking that she and her boyfriend could walk away from their responsibilities any day. In fact, they thought that they were doing a favour by giving up the baby for adoption. She was not even ready to marry her boyfriend and neither was she averse to continuing her relationship with him. One of my colleagues sarcastically remarked that probably they had come to rag us. I could understand one's tears, one's helplessness to be unable to keep their baby, but the coldness in her eyes infuriated me. It broke all my preconceived notions of a woman wronged.

A few days later, she had a friend from the hostel who came to take her home. We couldn't hold her back. She left the hospital without any remorse for the 'unclaimed baggage' that she was leaving behind, and one that she never came back to see. The hospital was left with no choice but to send the unwanted baby to the orphanage.

I was left with a strong sense of dismay. At least, the West was bold enough to acknowledge the changing moralities of their society. What had gone wrong here? Was it the deteriorating moral values, or lack of sex education and knowledge of contraception that made them behave like this? There must have been some lacunae in the healthcare system that led people to quacks. This was a failure of the whole system that a pregnancy went about without any check-ups and landed in complications? So many questions unanswered… so much to brood over…

I, who always thought of women as the silent sufferers, learned a new facet of womanhood. Yes, the world continues to spring surprises. And from every twist and turn, we come out just a little wiser. So was I, and still I had so much more to learn…

12
THE JOURNEY

"Hope sprouts green on the morning dew,
My branches wake up with life anew,
Rising sun after a tumultuous past
Happiness wakes my future at last ..."
(From my poem *The Naked Tree,* published in the book *Spectrum*)

'We can't continue this pregnancy!'

I looked at the determined faces of the couple sitting in front of me. Just a few days back, Kavya had looked so happy when the report read positive. Isn't pregnancy a natural culmination of a marriage? They had struggled so hard for the last two years to make their marriage work. Would this not make their relationship stronger? I looked with obvious reluctance at them.

Kavya said slowly, 'We don't want anything to come between us and our children.'

Her eyes darted anxiously to the two small boys playing outside the clinic. Both were around four years old. No, they were not twins, but brothers born only six months apart. Yes, they were step-brothers.

Aditya, who had been silent for a long time, intercepted quietly. 'It was not an easy decision, but then God has never made it easy for us,' he laughed.

I agreed with him. Life had not been a bed of roses for the two of them. They had sailed on a shaky boat, yet they had managed to stay afloat. I respected him above many people, for he had paid a heavy price to achieve that. Peace now replaced the lines of worry on his face. Once I had seen different emotions there – fear and anxiety. And that had mirrored on my face, too, as we stood helpless, watching life drain out slowly but surely from someone he loved and I had grown to admire.

The first time I had met Aditya was when he guided his heavily pregnant wife Urvashi into the labour room. She was having labour pains. His wife had been a regular patient at our clinic and we had all grown to like her a lot. Her quiet demeanour and soft voice had won our hearts. She was very beautiful, too. God had been kind to her, or that's what we thought. Her husband was posted outside and had come home just a week back to be with her. She stayed with his parents who took good care of her, but she always missed him. They made for a perfect picture together, and the handsome couple was an object of envy to many. He stood holding her hands as she laboured. Unlike a majority of women who howled in pain, she suffered quietly, not once letting her voice reach outside the room and disturb others. Her quiet dignity was almost ethereal. Soon, much to the joy of everyone, she delivered a healthy baby boy. It was almost midnight, but the night was far from over. The darkness of the long night was meant to engulf us.

Unexpectedly, Urvashi started bleeding. There were small tears which were oozing but we stitched them. She still kept losing blood. Post-partum haemorrhage, a known entity that threatens the life of a woman, cast a dark shadow over her. The very mechanism that prevented excessive loss of blood after delivery, went overboard and consumed the clotting factors, causing more bleeding. A dangerous play had started, with a brutal destiny. From giving blood products to giving fluids, from medicines to prayers, we tried all. But our every defence turned out to be a notch weaker than the offence that was mounting inside her body. As a desperate measure, we shifted her for surgery to remove the offending structure – her uterus. She was conscious when she was being wheeled into the theatre and two tiny drops rolled down her cheeks – the evidence of her silent agony. She held her husband's hands and didn't say anything.

She never recovered from the onslaught. Her husband and her family turned to stone as she lay, covered in white, with a thick veil of silence surrounding her. And I stood watching them, unable to reach out. Maybe we could have done this somewhat differently. However, my anguish, much like her, didn't make any sound. If only God didn't make us do his dirty job. We get the brickbats while he walks away with the accolades.

'You could not change our destiny,' a voice said, startling me.

It was Aditya who stood behind with folded hands. I had seen people creating a ruckus in hospitals in the grief, but here he was, thanking me, even as his world turned upside down. His humility touched me more than words can ever define and, strangely, left me feeling worse.

Two days passed before our neonatologist decided to call us. Nobody had turned up from the family to check the baby. The hospital had called a day before. Somebody had answered and promised to get back. However, even that was more than twenty fours hour now. Sometimes people held the unfortunate babies responsible for such tragedies and abandoned them, but somehow, in this case, it didn't seem true. I decided to call Aditya. He answered my phone and sounded really broken. In all the turmoil of the last two days, the baby had completely slipped from their minds. He was bewildered, and apologized profusely. The extent of their trauma was beyond imagination, and sympathy was a poor substitute. The next day, his parents came along with him and took the baby home. Every time Aditya looked at him, he was reminded of his broken dreams, and bittersweet memories rose to taunt him. But how could he blame an innocent baby who was now the only reminder of his wife? He owed it to her that their son should never feel the absence of his mother. And as he buried his head in his baby's soft skin, he could feel the warmth of his lovely Urvashi seeping in. From that day, he became both mother and father for the baby.

Life had different priorities now. He shifted back to Delhi, and the only time he left his son Rehan was when he had to go to the office. Rehan had become almost an obsession for him. His parents watched, worried, as he slowly withdrew into a shell. Urvashi's parents, too, clung heavily on to Rehan, for they saw their beautiful daughter live in him. Aditya had also grown very close to them. It seemed almost natural to presume that he would get married to Urvashi's younger sister but, unfortunately, she had already committed herself to somebody. Without disclosing anything to him, his parents started looking for someone who could be a mother to little Rehan, and a companion to the now reclusive Aditya.

An ordinary-looking Kavya had had a love marriage. She came from a wealthy family and fell in love with Kuldeep. Their parents had no objection and amidst a lot of fanfare, they both got married. However, two years down the line, she started feeling the pressures of having a child. Much to their disappointment, she couldn't conceive. After trying for almost a year, the desperate couple decided to go for an IVF (in vitro fertilization) pregnancy. They were blessed with a baby boy a year later and happiness touched the zenith. But strange are the ways of the Almighty. An unknown enemy in the guise of a mosquito bit her husband. He suffered from dengue and it proved to be fatal. Her world crumbled, and her pleas fell on the deaf ears of a cruel destiny. She was left alone, clutching her son who was not yet one year old, in her arms. Her father couldn't bear to see the sight of Kavya as she stood crying helplessly. He was worried about her future.

She was barely twenty eight, and a long life stretched out in front of her. It pained him to imagine her struggling alone all her life. Her vulnerability touched a raw point in his heart. He could buy everything for her but how could he make her lovely eyes smile? Kuldeep's pyre had not yet turned cold but his determination to make her live again was already strong.

Kavya was disgusted by her father. How could she accept anyone in Kuldeep's place? Yet as days went by, a strange loneliness filled her heart. She longed for someone to indulge her. She held her son's hands but missed his father on the other side. She missed his strong arms supporting her when she braved the rough realities of life. Her eyes searched for the absent Kuldeep everywhere, till tears blinded them. Kuldeep's parents were witness to her suffering and had no objection to her remarrying. They were more than happy to keep their grandchild. After all, he was the spitting image of their youngest and beloved son. But the mere thought made her clutch his fingers tighter. Bereft of his father, how could she deny a small child his mother, too? Fate had been cruel to her, but how could a mother be cruel to her son? Kuldeep might have deserted them but she would never desert his son.

Days passed by and her father discovered the hypocrisy that plagues the Indian society. It was no easy cake to marry off a widow. Previously unmarried guys were not even ready to consider her, and he purposely stayed away from them. All he could find were men who were either divorced, or widowers with a small child at home. Their demands were very simple. Their child wanted a mother, and they sought a companion. Kavya suited them but only on one condition. She could not bring her son along. Kavya shuddered as she listened to this. Men who cared so much about their own children were so ruthless towards her son. They demanded so much from her yet were not ready to give an inch. She felt insulted by the patriarchal mindset. She could never give Kuldeep's place to such unfeeling men who asked her, selfishly, to be a mother to their child, but abandon her own son.

She was better off alone than being with such people. Her father tried hard to convince Kavya to let go of her son, but she was not ready to compromise. Reluctantly, he was forced to accept the futility of his efforts. His hopes quashed, it marked the end to his dream of seeing her married again. However, every time one thinks that the end has arrived, life opens a new chapter ...

I was surprised to see Kavya sitting in my clinic. It had been more than a year that her son was born, and I knew about the tragedy that had struck her. She was having some vague complains and, as we talked, I saw her son sneezing a lot. He was not keeping well those days so I sent them both to the paediatrician. He was in his clinic just a few rooms ahead, and, after a while, as I passed his room, I was surprised to see Kavya's son Rohan playing with Rehan. It was always a delight to see Rehan. His father had gone to bring a candy for him while his grandfather kept a watch. I couldn't resist sitting with them. Rehan and Rohan looked almost like twins. Aditya returned and swooped his shrieking son up in the air, much to the awe of Rohan. At that point, Kavya came out of the doctor's clinic looking for Rohan who had quietly slipped out. She scolded him and, to her surprise, he burst out crying. Aditya stopped abruptly and lifted him in his arms, giving him a candy. Rohan stopped crying and blew him a flying kiss for his generosity. They made a cute picture and, for a moment, I could see Kavya watching him with a strange expression. However, it was over quickly, and I saw her thanking Aditya formally, before walking away with a reluctant Rohan dragged on his toes. Aditya moved inside the paediatrician's clinic with his son. His grandfather waited outside and was curious to know about Kavya and her sweet boy. As I narrated her tragic story, I saw his eyes fill with compassion. A secret thought lighted up his eyes.

I was surprised to receive a call from Aditya's father a few days later. He hesitated a little, before asking if I had any contact number of Kavya. Somehow, he was very taken by her and couldn't stop thinking about her. He wanted to talk to her family. I was pleased, even though I was not sure how Kavya's family would react. However, not deliberating much, I passed on her number to him. In the evening, Kavya's father called me up. He sounded excited and wanted to know all about Aditya and his late wife. I couldn't tell him much, but having seen him at a very raw phase, I could vouch for his dignity. My words were reassuring to him and he couldn't thank me enough. It was ironic that the hospital where they had lost everything, was now promising them a new life. Payback time, I wondered.

Aditya and Kavya were married in a simple ceremony in a temple, a month later. They had kept a small reception for their close family and friends. They were now parents of two small, but naughty, boys. Kavya had made special efforts to dress them up in the same clothes.

Their first priority, now, was to become good parents, and then good spouses. It was a difficult task. Rehan was used to being with his father and threw tantrums now that he saw so many people around him. Rohan was used to being pampered by so many people and suddenly found himself alone, with a mother who was busy looking after another boy and his father. And to make things worse, they fought a lot. At times, Kavya would break down. Days were traumatic as she struggled hard trying to prove herself to be a good mother, and nights were haunted by the ghosts of their past. Moreover, they now had four sets of parents to look after. The need to gradually wean off from the clinging grandparents, without traumatizing them, was a major roadblock in their growth as a couple. Ultimately, it was their perseverance that showed them the way, till one day, life was forced to smile down at them again. Kavya won over Urvashi's parents, and Aditya took the place of Kuldeep in his parents' heart...

Yes, they were a couple now. Their two sons completed their family. They didn't want anything to come between them – neither the memories of their past, nor the promises of a different future. I accepted that and wished them well.

Nothing lasts forever – neither your good times nor your bad times. Life moves on, undeterred. At some point, Kavya and Aditya were destined to meet. Kuldeep and Urvashi had accidently strayed into their lives, and were meant to be their co-passengers only for a short while. They were never their final destination in the journey of life.

And it was not yet over. A new journey had begun. The journey of Kavya and Aditya...

13
THE IRONY IN
THE LAND OF DURGA

"Amidst the festive splendour,
Throbs the underrunning bias.
Behind the bubbly kanjakas
Breathes their trauma and their trials.
The Mahisasurs still roam around free.
Oh the mighty Durga!
Why can't you feel
Why can't you see
The irony in the land of kanjakas..."
(Adapted from my poem Irony in the land of *Kanjakas*, published
in the book The *Dewdrops... a journey begins*)

She had been waiting for a long time. A battery of tests and
clearances from so many departments awaited her before she
embarked on her journey. She would suffer pain, but from her
pain, someone would get the gift of life. These patients always

invoked a sense of awe and reverence. They were healthy women, willing to undergo a major surgery and donate a vital organ, simply out of love and duty. I always made it a point to ask about the recipient. In this case, he was her sister-in-law's husband. What made her do this?

We don't have a choice. If I don't, he will die. Who else will do this?'

Yes, who else. For the last couple of years since the hospital started its transplant programme, I had seen many donors who were ready to walk over fire for their loved ones. A wife paying for the sins of a drunkard husband who lay helpless with liver failure, a mother... a daughter... a sister... I had seen them all. They were, in the majority of cases, women. The loss of a male member was unbearable. He had to be saved at any cost. The number of male donors was, ironically, scarce. Conspicuous by their absence, they got away under the guise of being the sole bread earners of the family. That made their lives more precious. And women indulged them, deliberately discouraging their male relatives. Another role was assigned to the woman, the nurturer, making her do what she was best at – giving life. Strangely, the society still didn't acknowledge their benevolence. It continued to shy away from accepting the compassionate girl child. Lord Ganesh – the first successful case of 'transplant' – smiled knowingly. He was *Siddhivinayak*, the God of wisdom. Why couldn't he impart some sense to the people of my country?

I had just delivered a woman's twin baby girls. She had been inconsolable since then. Embarrassed, her mother and mother-in-law were trying their best to calm her down. Somehow, her behaviour reflected on both of them.

Another patient underwent an emergency surgery because she was having uncontrollable bleeding, endangering both her and her baby's life. She delivered an 800-grams-preterm baby girl who had to be kept in the nursery, needing intensive care. Estranged from her husband, she carried on with this pregnancy much against the wishes of her parents, in the hope that it might bring back her wayward husband. It almost did that. Her husband and his parents came at the time of the surgery, blaming the hospital for conspiring with the patient's family and delivering a preterm baby unnecessarily. They were caught on CCTV, manhandling and pushing around the patient's father and uncle, as they were angry. The women in their family bore only sons, and they blamed the patient for giving birth to a girl. She had brought nothing but a 'burden' to the family. And they didn't think twice before abandoning the little, innocent bundle that lay helplessly in the nursery, unmindful of the injustice surrounding her. Shrugging off all responsibility, they were now untraceable. These were not cases in isolation, neither was it unusual to see people getting depressed over having a baby girl. Ironically, even the hospital bills were justified if they were blessed with a boy...

Breaking off from my pensive mood, I wished the generous woman good luck. She was gynaecologically fit for surgery. She had a whole lot of errands to complete before her surgery two days later, and I had a list of patients to see before I wound up.

As I turned to call the next patient, I noted some stocky men clad in stark white khadi kurtas sitting outside my clinic. I hoped they were not politicians. Politicians were a pain in the neck and I had neither the time nor the patience to cater to their whims. They didn't let me wonder for too long, and entered my room with folded hands. Looking at my raised eyebrows, one of them rushed to say, "We are the village elders of a small town in Haryana. We want your help. A case has been brought to our consideration by one of the families in the village. The son of that family isn't getting along with his wife. He has said that there is something wrong with her and she can't make him happy in bed. We want you to check what is actually wrong with her.'

This was so outrageous. Did everyone in the village know about their sex life? Suddenly, the room felt stuffed. 'So, they report everything to the village elders?'

'That's how it works in our village. We solve cases much quicker and are not as impersonal as the courts.'

The *khap panchayats*! So was I talking to one of those? But they didn't quite look dangerous. Maybe, we got biased by the media reports.

'We care for our people. We look after the interests of both parties.'

'Yet, you first wanted to check the "girl", and not the "son".' How objectionable it all sounded! Once again, the woman had to prove herself, not the man.

They were quick to refute it. They would definitely look into the allegation made by the girl, too.

I was still not very convinced about my role. As a doctor, I had limitations and certain boundaries I needed to respect. It was beyond my capacity to comment on any couple's sexual compatibility. It was something they needed to work out between themselves. A doctor could only look after the medical problems. We were not here to pass judgement on any woman, neither attest her sexual prowess. Moreover, I was bound by my professional ethics that required me to be discreet. But beyond everything, the mere thought of a woman being asked to prove herself to be sexually competent, sounded too humiliating, and disgusted me.

Obviously we were not thinking on the same wavelength. They looked puzzled.

'We assure you that there shall be no legal repercussions.' They didn't quite seem to understand what repelled me.

I had decided not to write anything out of context or not befitting a gynaecologist's prescription. They could make whatever they wanted of that!

The gentlemen moved out and a young woman in her twenties entered my room. She was accompanied by another woman, who I asked to wait outside. Her name was Munni and her discomfort was obvious. To an extent, it reflected on my face, too. I gave her a friendly smile before asking her if she had any complains. Tears welled up in her eyes but she simply shook her head in the negative. Her reluctance to talk was obvious and I was truly at a loss. I didn't want to sound curious or invade her already-exploited privacy, but there had to be some way around! After much deliberation, I wrote 'No gynae complains', and decided to complete the rest of my examination. There was nothing that suggested that she was in any way 'lacking as a woman'. She was co-operative enough.

I gently advised her, 'Maybe you could go for an ultrasound as part of a routine health check-up. That might actually prove to people that you don't have any abnormality internally, too.'

She simply broke down. Maybe she had been holding it for a long time.

Ma'am, please do not write anything that goes against me,' she pleaded, controlling her tears. 'My husband has never bothered much about me, but I still do not want to be dumped in this manner.'

She didn't appear to belong to this part of the country. Confirming my suspicions, she told me, 'I come from a small town in Jharkhand. I got married very young, barely out of my teens.' She continued, while sobbing, 'My parents died, leaving me alone. I was brought up by my uncle. One day, when I came back from school, my uncle told me that he had found a husband for me. I protested, but he remained unmoved. I just didn't want to marry. However, two days later I was informed that the groom's family was coming, and that I was to get married that day itself. I pleaded and cried, but he told me in definite tones that if I didn't get married I could leave the house. I had no choice. I came to this village in Haryana, a day later. My husband was much older than me. I discovered that many men had brought brides from other states because there were few women left of their own community. Maybe they had paid money to my uncle. I heard them calling us *molkis*. Though we were wives, yet we were more like unpaid maids whose sole duty was to serve the family and bear sons to their husbands.'

'How can one be sure to bear sons only?'

'They check with machines, and if it is a girl, they abort. We know we can bear sons only.'

'But sex determination is banned.'

'Perhaps in your city… but not in our village,' she told me innocently. 'Why want a girl, anyway? I would never want my daughter to suffer like me. I would rather have a son. He would at least protect me in my old age.'

From the eyes of the tortured woman, it sounded so justified. But how could I convince her that she was suffering a fallout of the skewed sex ratio, a consequence of this very mentality? These *molkis*, meaning brides who were 'bought', generally from other states, were a result of the rampant feticide in the state, leaving a sizeable population of eligible bridegrooms on a waiting list.

She continued, 'My husband was more cruel than my uncle. I slogged like a slave the whole day, but he was never happy. And he had a bad temper. I suffered his abuses, silently. However, things became worse when, even after two years, I failed to get pregnant. That made me useless in his eyes. He never took me to any doctor and simply assumed that I was barren. Then I heard rumours that he was having an affair with a girl from another village. He stopped coming near me, but my humiliation continued.' The black marks on her arms and back told me the horrifying tale of her agony.

She paused, and I listened, dumbstruck. Living in the safe confines of our home, we tend to imagine that such stories existed only in newspapers. And yet as I listened, I wished it desperately to be fiction, and not fact, crying in front of me.

'Since we came from a different state and culture, we were always looked down upon by everyone in the village. The circumstances in which I was brought here made me inferior to the brides from his own community, who had both the money and support from their families.'

Poor and illiterate, she allowed herself to be subjugated and exploited; denied even basic human rights.

'Could you not talk to anyone in the family?' I asked.

'There is hardly any female in the family. There's no sympathy from anyone. His mother is old, and thinks that the sun rises and sets with her sons. She never forgets to remind me that her son has spent so much on me. And according to her, being beaten up by a husband is just another wifely duty that I crib unnecessarily about. She relishes throwing my inadequacies at my face.'

'Inadequate? Of course you are not that!' It was difficult to hide my revulsion.

'Now that I am not useful to him, he wants to desert me. He has told his village elders that I am not good in the bed, either, and can't look after his needs as a man. Everyone was much too eager to believe him and brand me a failure. I tried to talk to my brothers-in-law. One of them is younger to my husband and had always been very kind to me, but for the last few days I am not too comfortable talking to him.' She stopped abruptly, not wishing to go on, but her eyes begged me to understand. A woman abandoned by her husband was an easy pick by any other man, especially in a town deprived of women. What kind of world was she living in?

It was better to divorce such a man, than keep living with him in such inhuman conditions. But where would she go? I had no answers to that. I finished writing my prescription. She had recovered her composure. Her elders walked inside. One of them asked me, suggestively, if everything was fine.

'Of course, she's a healthy woman. It's just that she has not been able to conceive. But that could be because of her husband, too. I have advised some investigations for both of them.'

They stared at me, looking slightly annoyed. They muttered a hasty 'thank you', before starting to leave my chamber. As they turned, I asked them, 'What are we doing about the disappearing girls in your village? Your village has the lowest sex ratio. Why are girls not born in your state?'

'We are looking into that. It is our top priority.' They spoke like true politicians.

We suffer, not because of our culture, but because of its false interpretations by such self-proclaimed culture guardians. Their gender-biased eyes can't see larger issues like domestic violence as they are only concerned with the petty domestic issues of people. Sadly, the focus is always on the one who benefits from the fire; rarely on the one who's consumed by it. And this village was no different in that regard.

'Please bring her husband next time, for the tests,' I said.

They looked bemused, yet nodded and left with Munni and the woman who had accompanied her. I knew I would not see Munni or her husband again. But in those few minutes, I had a close brush with reality. I had lived the irony that throbs through the land that worships Durga, but kills the *kanyas* (daughters)!

The day was far from over. I had some distressed patients in the ward. Well, I needed to tell them a little story. Leaving my chamber, I walked purposely towards the ward...

14
SOMETHING CALLED LOVE
- PART I

"I need to see the mirror,
I need to ride my terrors,
I need to break the trance,
I need to break this dance…"

It stung badly and she felt strangely wet. Sarika raised her hand to touch her ears tentatively, and froze. Her hand was dripping with fresh blood. Fear chilled whatever warmth was left in the room, and she shivered. As a gynaecologist, it was not an unfamiliar sight, and she always laughed when people asked her if she was ever scared of blood. However, for the first time, the sight of blood chilled her entire being. Her own blood! She tried desperately to shrug off the fear threatening to make her collapse. She had recently moved to this new city with her husband, Sarika thought bitterly. Who would she turn to? Before she collapsed, she called the hospital's emergency number. She worked there.

They promised to send the ambulance fast. Sarika had told them that she had met with an accident. She had not been very honest, but it shamed her to disclose the real reason. She sat on the sofa she had bought so lovingly just two days back. The warmth comforted her dazed senses a little, before she started hearing angry voices again. She pushed them away. She didn't want to listen to them. Should she call home? Her parents? Naah! She would break down and upset them. Her friends? They would be sleeping, considering the different time zone they lived in. They would ask too many questions. No. She would close her eyes and wait for the ambulance.

The red light twirled brightly over the loud siren of the approaching ambulance. The emergency staff rushed out and knocked at the doors. There was no response so they pushed it open. They entered cautiously, and stopped abruptly as they saw a bleeding Sarika sprawled over the sofa. They were well-trained in emergency procedures. Her pulse was a little feeble, but steady. Within minutes, fluid was rushing through her veins, and oxygen through her airways, and the ambulance was rushing back to the hospital, carrying with it a patient who had once been a doctor there.

Sarika woke up on a white bed in her own hospital. She felt a little bruised and light headed. The nurse gave her a welcoming smile. 'Good morning. How are you feeling, Dr Sarika? You have been lucky.' 'Lucky' was not the word she associated with herself, but still she smiled. She had been stitched and bandaged. The head nurse told her, 'Some nasty tears you had, in your earlobe, your nose, and above your eyebrows.' Were they getting suspicious? This was the third time she had come here. Soon, they would start doubting her frivolous injuries. Sarika had informed that she had slipped in her kitchen and hurt herself. If only she could be more honest. Any other woman living in this country would have complained the first time she was brought here. Was she ashamed, or was it guilt? Or was it simply an overriding feminine stupidity that thought she could still make it work. Tomorrow, she would sort things out. She felt too tired to think and turned her head away. A curtain divided her from the adjoining patient in the triage. It moved, and she caught a glimpse of a young woman on a ventilator. There were many white coats surrounding her. On one side stood a man holding the woman's blanched hands. Was he crying? Looked as if he was her husband. As she strained her head to see things clearly, she pressed on her injured ears and let out a painful cry. Immediately, the man pushed the curtains and leapt to her side. He held her hand firmly, and asked, 'Are you all right?' He could see there was no one with her. His warm hand reassured her, and Sarika felt strangely reluctant to let go. It was nice to feel the warm touch of a human being after a long time. He himself was grieving, yet he was so full of compassion. She wanted to say 'thank you' but could barely move her lips. A sigh escaped her, and with her hand still in the grip of the stranger, Sarika went to sleep.

Sarika was dreaming. She was arguing with her father. 'No, papa. This time I will not listen to you. Please let me decide.' Accepting that he had made a blunder last time, her father gave in. Sagar was handsome, and belonged to an affluent family. He was so suave and sophisticated. They had met through a matrimonial site. He was a management professional working in a corporate set-up. He made her feel wanted, and he wanted to know everything about her. She told him everything – the car she had bought, her investments, her savings till date, her salary. She didn't have anything to hide. She wanted to do it properly this time. He laughed at her choice of car and her investments, but she looked at him indulgently. With him beside her, she was not alone any more. She would now make the right choices. Her future would be secure. Sarika tossed uneasily on the bed and turned to one side. She saw herself getting married to him. Her red-coloured *lehenga* sparkled against his cream *bandhgala*. She was entering her bedroom decked with beautiful flowers. It was her wedding night. But where was Sagar? She strained to see him in the dimly lit room. Sagar was sitting on one side of the bed,

holding a glass of whiskey, looking lost and desolate. She came
near him and put out a hand to touch him. He recoiled. 'I love
Shreya,' he said. His first wife! She knew he had been divorced,
but he had never behaved like this. He was too drunk. To her
dismay, she noticed a line of pillows separating the two sides of
the bed. Her head whirled. How could fate be so cruel again?

The scene changed. She was talking to Shreya, his ex-wife,
who was his childhood sweetheart and his sister's friend. Shreya
was speaking bitterly, 'All he wanted was money. I got out of it as
soon as I realized. You do the same.'

'No. He loves you!'

'Grow up, dear. He loves no one.' Sarika didn't believe that.
She would make him love her.

The scene changed again. They were both trying to make
their relationship work. Sarika had handed over all her passbooks
and savings to him. She had accepted her bad business sense.
She was a doctor. She was supposed to have a lot of money. She
would sell that car, too, and give him the money. He smiled. They
came close. He wrapped his arms around her and kissed her.
Sarika was ecstatic.

Sarika was seeing something different now. She was six
months pregnant. She had suffered from pain and bleeding in
the early months. Yet, the baby was growing well. They were to
visit her friend who had come from India, today. She handed
over all her money to him. However, today she had got her
salary so she went and bought a smart cardigan for her friend.
But why was Sagar looking at her like that? He looked furious.
He was accusing her of being a spendthrift. Something inside her
revolted. She was earning, damn it! She slogged in the hospital
while he had left his job and was studying. Why couldn't she
buy something, once in a while? Sagar didn't like dissidence.
Suddenly, Sarika was reeling backwards. Had he hit her? Or
had he pushed her? Or both? She lost her balance and fell on
the floor. Sarika saw herself clutching her abdomen in pain. She
rushed to the hospital. Her baby girl was just 700 grams. She

was born distressed, as the placenta had separated during the fall and she had been cut off oxygen. Her poor baby couldn't make it. Sagar looked grim.

There were loosely-fitting scenes. Puzzled, like a jargon, she lived through them without understanding much – Sagar shouting at her; Sagar crying for his ex-wife; Sagar hitting her; blaming her for everything; asking for money, money and more money; Sarika reaching the hospital sometimes with a black eye, and sometimes with a twisted thumb. Sarika, the gynaecologist, or Sarika, the battered wife?

Then she saw her first sign of real defiance. Sarika fell in love with a sofa and she bought it. Her parents were going to come next month. But Sagar was so angry. He let out a string of profanities. Suddenly, not caring any more, Sarika went to her room. They were sleeping in separate bedrooms for a long time. She wanted to be out of this place for a while. She looked for her passport but couldn't find it. Sagar was not in his room. She searched everywhere and finally found it in his cupboard. As she turned, she saw Sagar standing near the door. He was accusing her of snooping in his room.

But why had he stolen her passport?

Because she was good for nothing. She could hardly take care of herself. She needed to be controlled.

Her patience snapping, Sarika reminded him that she was a doctor and earning for him, too. Sagar didn't take that kindly. He hit her, and hit her more every time she shouted back, until she collapsed.

He was the one who had brought her to this country. She was supposed to be thankful for that, the ungrateful wench!

Sarika was moaning in the bed, throwing away her sheets drenched in sweat. A nurse was shaking her, trying to wake her up. 'Dr Sarika, you are having a nightmare.' Sarika opened her eyes and looked at the nurse. No, it was not a nightmare. She was reliving the story of her life. But she couldn't tell her that. As she got up, she realized that she had been shifted to a private room. The nurse brought her some water and something to eat. Suddenly, she remembered the man who had held her hand so tightly. Warm blood gushed to her cheeks, in embarrassment. The nurse drew back the curtains, and bright sunlight filled the room with warmth. On an impulse, she asked the nurse who came to attend her, 'Who was that woman in the bed next to mine? What had happened to her?'

'You mean Mrs Tanya Sharma? She is sick, poor girl. Her heart is not working well and she is pregnant, too. By the way, her husband Subin came to see you once. He was asking about you.' Since both of them were Indians, the staff didn't think it was unusual.

A strange happiness filled Sarika's heart. It had been so long since anyone had shown concern for her. She didn't see Subin again, but on the day of her discharge, she saw a bunch of flowers in her room, with a small card which read: Smile through your tears and the world will shine with you. Sarika's lips lifted at the corners.

Not wanting to go back to her home and confront Sagar there, she took a cab to a friend's house. They were horrified to know about Sagar and advised her to report him to the police. It was high time she did that. Sarika got a restraint order issued against him, and he was forbidden to come near her. She moved to another house. When she went to the bank, she found, to her surprise, that all the money had been moved to his personal account. Her friends told her that he had sold most of the furniture, too, when she was in the hospital. Disgust rose like bile, in her blood. She had loved and lost again.

Such a 'once upon a time' thing, that something called love!

Her scarred past rose to taunt her, but she remembered a stranger holding out flowers asking her to smile, and she turned back. She should be immune to cruel men, anyway.

Like a phoenix she would rise out of the ashes, once again.

(To be continued...)

15
SOMETHING CALLED LOVE
PART II

"But a flicker and it was gone,
A veil so quickly, densely, drawn.
Strangers again, they sat forlorn;
She had lingered too long,
She had wandered too far,
Yet a door she left slightly ajar ..."

Sagar was not her first husband. Five years back, while doing her post-graduation, her father had called her home. That day she had met Tushar. His parents had a nursing home and he was an orthopaedic surgeon. It was a match made in heaven. They got engaged the next day, and a starry-eyed Sarika returned, wearing her heart on her sleeves. She could be seen hanging around the solitary telephone in the hostel, or waiting for his visit. Strangely, the calls were few and the visits none. On a few occasions that he promised to come, he didn't bother to turn up. No apology, no explanations! Strange behaviour from a recently engaged guy.

However, the eyes conveniently ignore what the mind doesn't want to see. She learned to live through his indifference, convincing herself that not all guys were demonstrative. Love ignores and forgives too. She got married a few months later.

Her marriage was a typical Punjabi affair. A youthful, 23-year-old waited for him on her wedding night, with dreamy eyes. However, her inscrutable groom continued chatting with his *bhabhi* (brother's wife), all night. She was fast asleep when he came back in the early hours of the morning. She woke with a start when he entered.

'I am tired,' he said brusquely, and turned his back.

That was supposed to be my line, she thought humorously, before going back to sleep again.

She played the adoring wife and, he, the aloof husband; always finding a reason to stay away. Thankfully, they were soon on their honeymoon. She was happy to be out with him alone at last, away from the 'omnipresent' *bhabhi*. Maybe she was getting jealous, but Tushar was always so attentive to his much older, and more beautiful, sister-in-law.

Her honeymoon was a bigger disaster than she could ever imagine. Her husband never showed any inclination to come close to her. Her every advance was scorned. If she tried to broach the subject, he would admonish her for thinking only about one thing. She was getting confused and upset. With a heavy heart and a suspicious mind, she returned back home with him. Something was definitely wrong. On coming back, he plainly told her that it couldn't work between them and she should leave. They called a cab for her, and in a haze she left home, leaving behind everything that was once precious to her, including her belongings. Her parents were shocked. They tried to mediate, but when her husband sneered about how unattractive Sarika was and how she failed to turn him on, they gave up. Sarika's life had plunged into darkness. A smart and intelligent doctor went on to buy books on personality development. Her repeated attempts at reconciliation were thwarted at every step by a hostile Tushar.

It started affecting her professional life, too. She was hell-bent on putting everything on stake for him, and he was hell-bent on ridiculing and destroying everything for her. She touched the lowest point of her life.

One day, after a lot of pressure from her friends, she decided to see a psychiatrist; of course, Tushar refused to go with her. They met the doctor, separately. She got a call from the doctor the very next day, asking her to get out of the relationship. It finally dawned on her that he was an insecure man hiding behind his own incompetencies. She had wasted five years of her life on an impotent man who refused to accept it. He didn't give her an easy divorce, either.

She now wanted to live again, and this time on her own terms. That was when Sagar came along. In her haste to do everything right, she made the same mistake. She let a man become her priority, again. Maybe she was fighting her destiny. Maybe she was trying to write her story on a wrong page. Finally, she would altogether tear off that page from the book of her life. She was a closed book for any man now, she vowed.

Sarika was learning to enjoy her own company. It was so much easier to fall in love with yourself – no expectations, no bitterness, no trauma of heartbreak. She had joined the hospital a week back, and was looking forward to hone her skills in infertility, a branch that fascinated her. She was on duty when she was surprised to see Subin, again. He had walked into the triage with his wife, who was in labour, and acutely distressed. Her already-weak heart was failing and she had to be kept in the ICU. Sarika delivered the small baby girl of Subin, and watched life slowly drain out of his wife's body. Something drew her towards him. The metaphors were striking. Subin had been rejected by life; Sarika had been rejected by love. Yet she held his hands, just as he had held hers. His daughter was critical and was kept in the nursery. Subin suffered the onslaught of the tragedy, silently. Who said life was kind? He knew about his wife's illness before their marriage, but he thought his love would win against all odds. The unplanned pregnancy had ruined the precarious balance her heart was hanging on to. He had wanted termination, but his wife hid the pregnancy till it was too late.

He bid adieu to a hospital which was witness to his tragedy. However, he carried the fragrance of the flowers that Sarika had sent him, with a small note: Smile through your tears and the world will shine with you. The memory brought a smile to his lips. He could sense that she had been suffering from a problem, and yet she was so caring. Blessed are some people. Strangely, he felt so protective about her.

The little girl, lying helplessly in the nursery, reminded Sarika of her lost dreams. She couldn't help visiting the nursery everyday to know about her well-being. At times she came across Subin, but other than the cursory hello, they hardly interacted. The nursery was going to be the baby's home for another two months.

Sagar still managed to create a ruckus in her life. He once broke the lights outside her porch, but the strict laws of this country made it easier to deal with him. There were times when she felt lonely. The empty house haunted her, and she took recluse in the virtual world. One day, she was surprised to see a friend request from Subin on a social networking site. She didn't hesitate in accepting it. They chatted for a while before she logged off.

Subin's baby had been discharged a few days ago. The nursery was going to miss her but was happy that she was finally going home. His sister had come along with him. He could barely manage here alone, so he was taking the baby to India. Life had different priorities now and he didn't want his daughter to suffer. He had a big family in India, and the baby could be looked after well. Subin was grateful to Sarika for all that she had done for him. Sarika smiled.

Life was moving on. Sagar was now receding as a distant memory. The unfairness of life hurt at times, but then she would think about the lovely things that made her happy, like the pictures

Subin sent of his daughter. He had named her Sarika. He wanted
her to become a generous doctor like her, he laughed, brushing
off her surprise. They had become good friends, and she used to
look forward to chatting with him. He had settled in India and
she missed baby Sarika. She had become so adorable. She was
crawling now, and Sarika longed to cuddle her.

It had been more than a week that she had spoken to Subin.
Sarika was getting jittery. She missed the baby's gurgling sound,
not Subin, she reminded herself. Maybe he was sick, or maybe
the baby was not keeping well. She texted him but he didn't reply
to any of her messages. Sarika was now as anxious as she was
angry. It was fine; anyway, he was not bound to talk to her.

She was about to go to sleep when her phone beeped. Her
mood lifted, and she felt strangely happy. He had sent her a
simple 'Hi'.

She planned to ignore it, but instead sent: 'Where have you
been?'

He just sent a smiley. She disliked emoticons.

She was getting angrier, when he sent: 'Was out with friends.
Bad signal there.'

I bet, she fumed. 'Friends, or girlfriend?' she asked.

'Girlfriend!'

She didn't like that at all. She stared at the phone for a long
time, and then wrote 'Go to hell'. Let him make out whatever he
wants of that.

He laughed back: 'Hahaha! Jealous, are you?'

He must be out of his mind! She wrote back: 'I don't need to.'

'Hmmm… did you miss me?' He was acting strange, but she
liked the teasing Subin.

'Like a hole in my head.'

She smiled, and then on an impulse she wrote back: 'I missed
Sarika.'

He replied: 'I missed her too.' She was not sure which Sarika
he meant, but she went to bed with a little smile hovering around
her lips. That day marked a new beginning in their lives. Suddenly,

they wanted to talk more, share more. Maybe they both were trying hard to leave behind their past. With clenched fists he listened, when she told him about her two husbands. He wanted to kill both of them. The intensity of his own anger shocked him. He didn't want her to be hurt again. Sarika was coming to India and he wanted everything to be perfect for her. They planned to meet in Goa. The romantic beaches of Goa added fuel to their feelings. They spent days and nights, lost in each other. Sarika had never been happier. She felt heaven in his arms. It didn't matter if it was lust; she didn't want to love. At least, there was truth in lust. Love didn't last. She believed only in lust.

It was bliss, but something troubled her. Subin belonged to a very different culture and was much younger to her. And yet, these differences didn't matter to him. Subin wanted more. He wanted marriage and children. Sarika never wanted to walk those roads, again. They had their first fight, that day. Subin didn't understand why she treated him as if he was good for only one thing; Sarika wanted nothing more from him. She wanted to keep him closely guarded, like a secret mistress; Subin wanted to flaunt her to the whole world. He didn't want to be her cheap little secret; she didn't want people to laugh at her, again.

Sarika cried, 'Why can't we just have an affair?'

He had to give in, and reluctantly agreed to accept her on her terms. He promised to make no demands to make their relationship permanent. Sarika was happy, but felt strangely let down by his acceptance. They spent golden nights in each other's arms. Soon, it was time for her to go back home. They promised to stay in touch and, with a heavy heart, Sarika left India.

They moved into different hemispheres, yet tried to snatch time together, whenever possible. Talking to him was becoming a habit she tried hard, but failed, to break. However, lately, Subin had become a bit vague. She hoped everything was fine. He evaded her questions, but then his passion would make her forget everything. After all, that was what she wanted, isn't it? Her spirits lifted when he told her that he was going to come to see her soon. He had promised to bring baby Sarika, too. Things were going just as she wanted, until one day, she saw his picture online. He was smiling, with his arms around a pretty girl. As she scrolled down, she saw many congratulatory messages. She was aghast. How dare he?

Subin was surprised to hear from her. She rarely called. Maybe she wanted to deny him any real contact. Talking breaks the elusions of texting, and she wanted to remain elusive. She came straight to the point – 'Who is she?'

'Oh, my parents have found a girl for me. They said they were getting old and couldn't be burdened with baby care, any more.'

'How could you?' Sarika cried.

'How does that affect us?'

'It doesn't? How can you even say that?'

'Oh, we can carry on our affair. No one will know!' Subin sounded so insulting.

'You are so bloody cheap.'

'But then, that's what you wanted, isn't it?'

Go to hell! Sarika slammed the phone down and broke into tears. She had done it again. Against her better judgement, she had let a man wreck her life, again. She should have known that Subin would not live on her terms, all her life. But isn't this what she had asked him to do?

She wept for herself. This time, it was her own insecurities that had destroyed everything.

She woke to the sound of the doorbell ringing. She didn't want to talk to anyone. But somebody was really persistent. She thrust open the door and was dumbstruck to find Subin standing outside, with flowers in his hand. She was about to slam the door, when Subin came in and prevented her from closing it.

She must have wept all night, yet she looked so beautiful. Subin could have kicked himself for hurting her. She was so stubborn. What else could he do? Silently, he gave her the flowers. There was a small card tucked inside: Smile through your tears and the world will shine with you. On reading that, Sarika burst out crying. She couldn't help it.

She hardly realized that Subin was taking her into his arms, stroking her hair, and saying sorry, again and again. She stopped crying as soon as realization hit home. She drew back, mumbling something incoherent.

Subin said, 'Isn't this what you wanted all along?'

Sarika looked miserable. 'I don't know what I want any more.'

Subin looked grim. 'I just wanted you to admit that you care for me more than you admit. All that stuff online was just a drama. It was meant to shock you out of your stupor. I have taken a big step risking everything and moving back here for you.'

Sarika watched him through a haze of tears, when realization struck. Hope was opening dreamy eyes in her heart, again. Subin gently asked her, 'Now Sarika, will you put us both out of misery and say yes?'

'Yes to what, Subin?' Sarika teased, as she kissed him on his lips.

Subin arms tightened in response, 'When you say yes to me, it'll mean everything to me. Though I don't mind if you have anything else on your mind.'

Sarika laughed, and it was a long time before either of them could talk.

The most unplanned thing, love! You don't find love, love finds you. It meets you at the most unlikely places, places as queer as hospitals. It comes looking for you, when you are looking elsewhere. It still makes the world go round, that something called love!

16
THE SPURIOUS IDENTITY

*"You want to look at the stars
but not the sky,
I dare to live,
Please look into my eyes ..."*

My younger son was unusually quiet that day. I hugged him, but he remained as morose as ever. Even the cartoons on the television could not pull him out.

'Hey babes, what happened?' I cradled him in my arms.

'He is such a baby, such a sissy!' his 'know-it-all' elder brother added, cynically.

'I am not girlish!'

That jibe brought some reaction from the dejected child lying in my lap. 'You saw that, mom. He even calls me gay! Just because I put my arms around him when I am sleeping...'

'What is gay?' I squealed in surprise. I was so careful to avoid the word whenever the kids were around.

'When boys like boys, and not girls. And you know, they even get married to each other.' He took pride in his knowledge.

'Really?'

'And it's illegal in India, though not in the USA,' he boasted, uninterrupted.

'How do you know that?'

'You yourself tell us to read the newspapers,' he looked at me irritatedly. 'Mom, you are getting menopausal.'

'Now what's menopausal?' I was ready to hit the roof.

He had the grace to look embarrassed. 'Actually, the other day you were telling aunty that your head of department is so irritating, forgets everything, and keeps snapping at everyone unnecessarily. Aunty said that she must be getting menopausal.'

I fumed, but could only say, 'You should never eavesdrop.'

'And you call him a baby' his elder brother suddenly quipped in. 'Babes, tell us what happened in school today. Did you fight with your girlfriend, or hey, was it a boyfriend?'

The two brothers were at loggerheads, again. Seriously! One child made you a parent; two a referee! It was useless to talk sense to either of them. Leaving them at their squabbling best, I started for the hospital. The changing times we live in… How easily this generation had accepted the changing norms of our society.

I was reminded of an old lady who had visited me the other day. She stood awkwardly in front of my clinic, looking a little unsure.

'You wanted to consult me?'

She just stared at me.

'You have some problem?'

She still kept quiet. Exasperated, I looked around.

'Actually, ma'am, she wants to talk to you,' a high-pitched voice interrupted. I noticed a thin boy who suddenly appeared at her side. He had long hair that bounced around his soft, delicate face. He had a feminine voice, and I noticed the bright nail paint he was wearing. My son would have called him a sissy, too, I thought humorously.

'*Beta*, I want an advice.'

I waited for her to elaborate.

'Well, I have heard that these days you can change the sex. Can you change a boy into a girl?'

Startled, I looked at the boy.

'Oh no, it's not him. Somebody wanted to know.'

I knew how much it must have cost her to come and speak to me. I didn't want to embarrass her. 'Not always. You will have to talk to a cosmetic surgeon. It's a long procedure… many sittings… not easy at all. It involves a lot of counselling before you are even considered fit to go through it.'

'What choice do I have?' she mumbled to herself. I pretended not to hear.

'It's expensive, too. And no, I don't know the exact amount,' I added, before she could interrupt.

Thanking me, she left, followed by her son. I wondered how she had come to terms with the altered sexuality of her son. There was a time when these topics were never broached in public. But thankfully, though it still carried a stigma, we were at least talking about it.

A woman's soul trapped in a man's body! That's how a friend had once described himself as he unsuccessfully tried to hide his anguish. Needless to say, he went on to marry under family pressure, ended up having children, too, and then the whole family got embroiled in an ugly divorce. It was difficult to pinpoint the culprit, but each one of them had been a victim. Living together, both he and his wife had become suicidal. Only time would tell what scars they had invariably given to their children. Strangely, his parents had yet to accept his sexual orientation and, somehow, still blamed his wife.

The untimely squabble between my children had made me late. A patient of mine was in labour. Making way through the anxious relatives, I reached her. She was not doing very well in labour, and suddenly, the baby's heartbeat started dipping. A decision for an emergency caesarean section was made, and the patient was quickly shifted to the operation theatre. All else was forgotten – even my forever-at-war children, at home – as we focused completely on taking out the baby. Soon, our efforts were rewarded by its loud wail. Nothing makes the team inside the theatre 'happier', than the 'cry' of a baby.

'Ma'am, is it a boy or a girl?'

It was a girl, but then it was not the right time to tell the patient. Who knows what effect it would have on her psyche?

'Sorry dear, we didn't see that. Let the baby's doctor come and tell you that.'

'OK, tell us what do we have here?' A little later, the paediatrician had the baby brought near her, draped in a sterile sheet, exposed just enough to make out its sex.

The patient squealed in delight, 'It's a girl! My baby, so sweet! Ouch! Is she the one who kept kicking me from inside? Thank you so much, Ma'am!'

She touched the baby in wonder, and kissed her. As the surgery was still going on, her hands were not free, and she could hardly do more than that. We had been through this so many times, but it never failed to lift our spirits. A baby is a sign that, despite all the turbulence, humanity is still alive.

'I hope nobody is going to be upset at home, now that it's a baby girl?'

'No, ma'am. We always wanted a girl.'

Thank God for that.

Relaxing a little, we went about finishing the surgery. The baby was now carrying an identification band around her wrist. It was a necessity, considering people blamed the hospital for having swapped their babies after delivery. Of course, the majority didn't have a problem if they had a baby boy.

It was almost six in the evening when I came out of the surgery. I noticed a flurry of activity outside another theatre. An excited staff informed me that a sex transplant surgery was going on. My curiosity took me into the theatre.

'Hey, what brings you here? Must be doing a caesarean,' the cosmetic surgeon called out to me.

'Well, not everybody does interesting stuff like you guys.'

He smiled at that.

'What are you up to?' I tried to peer into the operative field, not making much sense of it.

'I am making a penis,' he boasted. 'A functional one at that.'

My eyes went rounder and rounder. He laughed at my expression and went on describing, in detail, how he had made that possible.

'Yuck!'

'You say that! You don't understand her trauma. We have been working on her for about two years. So many stages. We removed her breasts, then her uterus and ovaries, and finally we are making her – err – him a man.'

'What's wrong in being a woman? Any day, a hundred times better than being a man.'

'I agree. You are better being a woman,' he teased.

I gave him a nasty look. They had been working since morning. It was not easy transporting so many nerves and vessels and they even took meal breaks in between. I seriously wondered what drove them to undertake such gigantic surgeries.

'It's a challenge,' he said to my receding back. Meeting challenges, or breaking nature's law? Whatever! He was welcome to take his challenges. I was happy doing my little job.

I was about to wind up, when my phone beeped.

'Ma'am, there is a strange patient in the casualty,' said the troubled voice of my resident doctor.

'What's wrong with her?'

'She has been brought by her husband. She has a very resistant high blood pressure, and some salt imbalance.'

'What's strange about that? Does she have a gynae complain?'

She sounded a little uncomfortable, 'Actually, the physician felt that he was not sure about her.'

'They are never sure about anything!' I couldn't resist adding, sarcastically.

We both reached the casualty together but could not locate the patient. The nurse looked at us understandingly, and led us to the bed of a tall, bearded man.

'Sister, we are from the gynae department!' My impatience was beginning to show.

'Madam, she is your patient,' said the casualty nurse, smiling a little.

'But, this is a…!' We stopped ourselves and looked at the records.

She was a 40-year-old man – sorry, woman – married for around fifteen years. She had always been hairy, but lately, it had become especially troublesome. She never took any treatment for that or went to any beauty parlour. Only her younger sister was allowed to shave her. Since the last few days she had not been well, hence her overgrown moustache and beard. She had always had a masculine appearance as far as she could remember, and strangely, she had never had her periods, either.

'Didn't you ever see a doctor for that?'

'I was scared, and so were my parents.' She lowered her eyes.

She indeed had little feminine assets.

'Your husband?' I suddenly remembered.

'I was good in studies and in sports, too. My husband is also a sportsperson and we had had a love marriage.' She looked at our raised eyebrows, and went on, 'We've had a normal relationship, madam. My husband is a very caring person. He never stressed about not being able to have children, and has always been very supportive.'

'You are indeed a very lucky person.' Hopefully, she hadn't noticed my omission; I had not called her a lucky 'woman'. 'And I must remember to meet this gentleman.'

Further examination confirmed our suspicion that she had ambiguous genitalia. There was a small indentation in place of the vagina, or a 'blind vagina' as we medically classified it. The rest was difficult to define. An intersex, is that what she was?

She had been brought up as a woman. Should we attempt to redefine her as a man when neither she nor her family was demanding us to? Why create psychological havoc by reorienting her sex, when she was well adjusted in her life?

My phone rang once again. 'So what do you think?' the physician sounded excited.

'I'm not sure. You would be doing an ultrasound. Let me know.'

Merely speculating is never the right course, especially in sensitive matters. Avoiding the curious and questioning glances, we left silently.

The next day brought some good news, and some bad news as well. Her ultrasound showed a big adrenal tumour. It must have been present for a long time, explaining her androgenic problems. It was secreting an overdose of hormones, especially the male ones, leading to her masculine appearance. The good thing was that she had a small uterus, and ovaries too, but they were probably not functioning because of the high level of androgens. No male gonad, or testis, could be found. The tumour didn't explain her blind vagina, but then it was seen in many normal girls, too. However, it did explain the ambiguous genitalia, to an extent. Probably she wouldn't need a redefining of her sex, but that still needed to be confirmed. They were planning the removal of her tumour, and hopefully, many of her symptoms would get better.

I met her worried husband who listened intently while we explained her condition to him.

'I have no problems with her physical appearance. I just want her to be well soon.' He looked indeed very much in love with his wife.

'Would you like to have a karyotype?' This was the only test that could prove conclusively that she was a woman, and not a man.

He pondered, discussed with his wife, and agreed. Maybe, they wanted to remove the nagging doubt they must have been carrying subconsciously. The tests were done, and the woman operated upon. The last I saw her, she was recuperating in the post-operative ward.

I was pleasantly surprised to see the couple, about six months after the surgery, in my clinic. Yes, she was a beautiful woman, though she had never been less in the eyes of her husband. But now, she wanted to feel wholesome. An incomplete feeling had been with her for a long time. People had judged them based on her looks, and even questioned their sexual orientation. It had made them reclusive, but all that was a thing of the past, now.

'There were times when I had started believing that I was neither a man nor a woman,' she admitted. 'My parents didn't want me to see a doctor because they were scared the *hijras* (transgenders) would take me away. My friends would often tease me about my appearance, and I always lived with a nagging fear. I had lost my self-respect. But then I met my husband. With his love, I learned to live again... but it is still a cruel world outside. I couldn't help feeling guilty for him. There were times when I would be flooded with fears, and doubt everyone, including my husband. Maybe that's the reason we agreed for the chromosomal studies. But he's truly been my anchor.' She looked at her husband with pride.

She hesitated a little and asked again, 'Can you make me a woman in the true sense?'

She wanted vaginal reconstruction, and correction of the altered anatomy of her genital system.

'It is plausible and not a very uncommon surgery. And once that is complete, your hormones could be checked, and maybe your physiology could also be corrected,' I said.

The road was long and tough, but she was fortunate to have her husband on her side at every step.

They left with dreams of a happy future. As I left for home, I could only imagine the trauma they must have endured at the hands of an unsympathetic society. If only we had a better support system, she might not have missed out on all those years. The story could have been completely different if her parents had brought her to a doctor back then. Lost in my thoughts, I didn't realise the traffic signal had turned red. I applied the brakes and the car stopped abruptly. Soon, a hefty man dressed in a woman's dress, started knocking at my window. I stared at him, or – hold on – was it a 'her'? Sighing, I turned away. The traffic light had thankfully turned green again...

17
THE CONDEMNED HUSBAND

"The scars of past run quite deep,
Pretensions are sometimes hard to keep,
And words tear the soul like a shark.
How I wish I had not seen,
The stranger shouting in the dark ..."
(From my poem *Stranger Shouting in The Dark*, published in the
book *Dewdrops... a journey begins*)

A call from the medical administration in the wee hours of
morning! Not the kind of emergency you expect to wake up to.
A couple had fought, and the wife threatened to jump from the
fourth floor. The hospital security was frantic. The situation was
tense, but under control. I absorbed it all through my sleep-dulled
senses. The patient Kusum was admitted under my care, with
premature labour pains.

The distraught ward nurse was waiting for me. She looked at
me accusingly, and took me to the patient's bedside with obvious
misgivings. A look at the couple, and I could gather the barrage

of emotions that must have kept them hostage all night. Kusum's eyes appeared red, and her face, puffy. I felt a familiar anger rising. When will men stop abusing their wives? I turned towards the husband who was sitting on the couch, head bent.

'What did you want to prove? What kind of a man hits a woman in this condition?'

From the corner of my eye, I could see the nurse say something. The husband rose, surprised. However, not in the mood to be interrupted, I went on rebuking him, 'You should be thanking your stars that we have not reported you to the police.'

Kusum was admonished, too, for behaving irresponsibly by trying to take her life. They had created unnecessary ruckus.

The husband finally managed to break through my well-meaning speech.

'She hit me!'

I could see the effort he put into saying that. Startled, I looked at the nurse, who nodded silently. Kusum bowed her head, and looked away. I was suddenly short of words. There must have been some provocation! Women don't hit their husbands! I tried to justify myself. Her husband went on to add that she always lost her temper very quickly. Things had become worse now, but he was tolerating only because of her pregnancy. I had the grace to look embarrassed. I mumbled, 'This is a hospital and you both need to behave like grown-ups.' It was all that I could manage.

A lot had changed. Roles had been reversed and my tone had lost the edge. I asked the husband to wait outside, and examined the patient. She appeared to be agitated, but stable. Being an admitted patient, she definitely had an advantage.

Her husband was waiting to talk to me. My hasty outburst had put me on the wrong footing, and I looked rather apologetic.

'Madam, Kusum has always been like this. My mother stays with us, and that is the bone of contention. My mother is also brash, at times, but I can't turn my widowed mother out of our home. Today, Kusum went too far and abused her in front of me. My mother broke down, forcing me to react. I am ashamed that

I momentarily forgot I was in the hospital and lost my temper.
But Kusum was also in no mood to tone down. She raised her
voice, and in the heat of the moment, hit me. When others tried
to intervene, she threatened to commit suicide.' He showed ugly
marks of violence on his body.

I didn't want him to clarify anything nor did I want to upset
a volatile patient who was pregnant. Sometime back, another
patient, after a verbal spat with her husband and mother-in-law,
drank a bottle of disinfectant and was brought to the hospital,
pregnant and critical. I wondered what made some women
behave like this. What the couple needed was good counselling
and some introspection. They needed to sort out the mess they
had made of their lives.

Next morning, much to our surprise, the couple was sitting
together amiably, with no traces of the storm of the previous
day. One marvelled at the flexibility of human emotions. It was
the patient's birthday that day and her husband had gifted her a
beautiful diamond pendant. No wonder they called diamonds a
woman's best friend! I hoped it would bring them peace as well.
The hospital would rather not be a witness to their domestic
turbulence again. Her pains had subsided and she went home.
Strangely, she never spoke about the incident. The husband on
his part looked apologetic and kept blaming his wife's hormones
for her unprecedented behaviour. We simply prayed for their
truce to last forever.

Another patient with severe pain in the abdomen was wheeled
into the hospital. She was doubling up in agony. Neeta, a 24-year-
old woman had been married for only a few months. A melee of
over-anxious relatives from both sides surrounded them. Despite
strict rules, people invariantly managed to bribe their way through
the hospital's security. A harassed-looking guy, whom I presumed
to be her husband, was sitting quietly, pushed to one side. The
relatives had to be forced outside, amidst obvious reluctance.

A tubal pregnancy or a twisted ovarian cyst was the most
probable diagnosis. The husband was called in to be explained.

However, soon the patient's mother barged in. She looked obliquely at the husband and he shrivelled.

'A pregnancy is out of question, ma'am' she hissed, as if the mere thought was repugnant to her. The patient, too, was not ready to entertain any doubts about pregnancy. On the contrary, the slightest mention of pregnancy brought a smug expression on the face of the husband. It was difficult to comprehend them. Steering clear from their family drama we asked for a blood test to rule out pregnancy, and an ultrasound of her abdomen.

The patient clenched her teeth in pain once again, before letting out an anguished, 'He can't!'

I turned, surprised, towards her. Her mother took me to a side and spoke in hushed tones, 'My son-in-law is a very simple person. I have nothing against him or his family. We have known them for a long time, but I have brought up my daughters in an unorthodox way. I have taught them the basics of life. Just after her marriage, when she came back home, she was always so tired.' Her mother looked at me suggestively.

I was at a loss to understand her. Looking at my bewildered expression, she nudged me, 'Her husband is only interested in listening to *bhajjans* (devotional songs) and fails to perform his husbandly duties.'

Their disappointment was understandable – but, tiredness? For all my medical experience, I could not correlate the two. However, I could now understand the hostility between the two sides of the family. Something personal between a couple had become a public discussion here. The husband still hovered around. I couldn't help feeling a tinge of sympathy for him.

Neeta was wheeled into the ultrasound room. A twisted ovarian cyst glared from the ultrasound machine, demanding urgent surgery. Much to the embarrassment of the patient and her family, the result was positive for pregnancy, too. The husband, with a new-found confidence, now came forward to discuss the case. A surgery in the presence of pregnancy had serious implications and he didn't want to take any chances. But for the patient Neeta, a pregnancy made false all her insinuations on her husband's incompetency. However, they didn't have much choice, as surgery was imperative. The operation went smoothly and the cyst was removed. It was too early to comment on the viability of pregnancy.

Neeta recuperated well after surgery. Her husband stayed by her side and appeared quite concerned. She gradually opened up and told me, 'My husband is a very spiritual person, not in the least inclined towards the physical aspect of a relationship. That makes me feel so rejected. I yearn for the love I deserve as his wife, but try as hard as I might, I always fail. The few desperate times that we were really together failed to fulfill me, and that further weakened his confidence. We are yet to have the physical proximity we should have as a couple. With every passing day, he has grown more aloof, and I, more depressed. When I went to my parents' place shortly after my marriage, my younger sisters and friends started teasing me. The tension of the past days surfaced and spilt over. I broke down under their questioning glances. My family members were naturally very upset. However, I am still hopeful. Maybe I could still make things work.'

This pregnancy had come as a surprise. Her frustration was understandable. It would have made more sense if they had worked on their marriage before getting pregnant. I could see that Neeta's family wanted an abortion but they were a little short of demanding it.

A week later, they came back, with the husband trailing behind. A repeat scan showed a pregnancy, but unfortunately, not a viable one. She needed a termination. Both sides of the family were, for once, united in grief. Human psychology is strange! Till the other day, she couldn't hear of being pregnant, but now she wanted it desperately. However, once again, life gave her no options. She underwent an abortion the next day. I advised her to first bring some order into her relationship before planning any future pregnancies. She just laughed bitterly at that. Her mother came into my chamber and once again regretted her son-in-law being a little illiterate in those 'special' areas. I appreciated the frankness Neeta enjoyed with her mother, even though it was apparent that it embarrassed her son-in-law.

A few days later Kusum was back in the hospital with labour pains. It was an effort keeping her quite. We were stumped by the abuses she hurled out at her husband and mother-in-law. Both of them scurried off. We understood the husband's reluctance to be a part of the birthing process, and allowed him to wait outside. Once there was a patient whose husband kept on pouring expletives, all the while his wife was in labour. He later explained that he was just trying to reach out to her. Well, he did manage to make the atmosphere light and us more literate in the common abuses of the day. Meanwhile, Kusum continued with the barrage of name-calling, directed at the two pitiful creatures waiting outside. Her husband was responsible for all her pain and deserved every bit of it. There was no love lost with her mother-in-law either, so she might have it as well. We reeled under the implied justification.

Finally, the tension of the labour room broke with the shrill cry of a healthy baby girl. The sight of the wailing baby made her suddenly quiet, and a tender smile lit her face. Soon, all grievances were forgotten and the whole family was united in celebrations. I marvelled at the strange psyche that plagues Indian families. Too many people; too much drama. But yes, things were never boring in our great Indian joint family.

In my mundane routine, I had forgotten Neeta, till one day she appeared before me looking depressed and withdrawn. Almost a year had passed since I had last seen her.

She told me sadly, 'Our relationship is not going anywhere. Most of the time, he is preoccupied with the *sadhu mandalis* (congregations of holy men). He even forces me to accompany him sometimes. And now to make matters worse, our relatives have started pestering me for a child. Who knows, it might just solve things between us! But how do I have a baby?' Her eyes clouded with sheer frustration.

She went on, 'I have tried everything – all in vain. And he refuses to take any treatment. If I persist, he accuses me of being obsessed with sex. All this is making me suicidal.'

In desperation, she had even tried to inject semen inside her through a syringe, but that didn't make her pregnant either. She now wanted an artificial insemination.

I was horrified! 'You first need to straighten out your life before putting a child into all this mess!'

She pleaded, but I remained adamant. Reluctantly, she had to drop the idea. I promised to help her husband get treated, but needless to say, he never turned up.

About two months later, I was met in the clinic by a radiant Neeta. Yes, she was pregnant. Looking at my raised eyebrows, she laughed, 'I tied him to the bedpost.'

I couldn't help smiling back, but I had a nagging suspicion that she had got an artificial insemination done somewhere. However, that was none of my business and I kept quiet about it. Her pregnancy went on smoothly. Her husband often came along with her. At the end of nine months, she was blessed with a baby girl. For the first time, she looked content. Shouldered protectively by her husband, she walked out of the hospital a few days later carrying the small baby nestled in her arms.

I passed her quite a lot of times, sitting in front of the paediatrician's clinic. Her gurgling baby was always a delight to look at. Apart from a casual greeting, we didn't interact much. Once I met her mother who, after a loud hello, went on to tell me that Neeta was staying with her these days. She didn't elaborate much and I didn't enquire either. There was nothing unusual about a woman staying with her mother after delivery, and I didn't give it much thought.

One day, I got a call from the medical records office informing me that a patient's husband, whose wife had delivered a year back, wanted a copy of her hospital papers. The administration was concerned if there had been any irregularities in the case.

Living in the days where a legal suit is filed at the drop of a hat, I requested to talk to him first.

I was surprised to see Neeta's husband walk into my room. He stood uncertainly, before I asked him why he wanted the papers. A little hesitant, he confessed that Neeta had filed for a divorce. He added bitterly that her mother was always interfering in their family matters. Instigated by her, Neeta kept cribbing about his simple lifestyle and was never satisfied with him. He was a deeply religious person, and she had never liked that. They had now filed a case of domestic abuse. They had also charged him for being impotent. I stared at him. He pleaded with me, 'Madam, you know very well that Neeta has been pregnant twice. I want the papers from the hospital to prove that. You can always testify in the court, as you were her obstetrician.'

I hated courtroom dramas. I told him firmly that he was welcome to use the hospital papers but it was onto his lawyer to prove things. I wanted to stay out of any legal mess.

He had always been a timid man and didn't protest much. I watched his retreating steps, not knowing which side my sympathies lay with. A toothless baby smiling through her shiny curls entered my mind, and in my heart, I knew where my loyalty lay. The poor baby had arrived on a boat that had lost its anchor...

A gentle nudge on my shoulder brought me back to the reality. Chanda, our OPD nurse, sounded excited. 'Ma'am, Babulal has come with a new bride again.'

I slumped on my chair, clasping my head in my hands. Babulal had become a habitual groom. Having a zero sperm count, he could never become a father. The first time he was told that, he went to his village and got married again. And with a new wife, he also changed his doctor in the hospital. This was his third wife and I was his new doctor.

I fumed inwardly, but then, patience is a virtue doctors rely heavily upon. I asked them to come in. Another story in the making! Just another day in the life of a gynaecologist...

18
A PHANTOM PREGNANCY

"A women labouring
in agony and pain,
What was she here to gain?
Holding her tears!
A result of love,
or deceit that cost her dear?"
(From my poem *Love's Labour*, published in the book *Dewdrops…*
a journey begins)

'We assist God in creating life' – the irony glinted outside the clinic. God silently mocked our efforts, even as we chased the forbidden dreams of many desperate couples, till he relented.

A villager had travelled a long way to reach this clinic. His wife had conceived many times, yet by some strange twist of fate, the ultimate bliss eluded them.

We were suddenly taken aback. Spread outrageously all over her perineum (the area between the anus and the vulva) was something suspicious, almost like vermillion and ash. The wife feigned ignorance about them, but the husband reluctantly admitted about seeing a *tantric*. They were trying to invoke the spirits. The vermillion and the incense sticks were part of some black magic they practiced. Thankfully, she had not got burnt.

The myths in the land of the snake charmers and skull worshippers, rose tauntingly. There were incidents of appeasing the spirits with blood and sometimes human sacrifice, too. A wild jungle sleeps in desperate minds. There are no rules here. Lines are drawn, yet boundaries are crossed. Can illiteracy and ignorance truly excuse such horrific behaviour?

'My ancestors, from the land of the dead across the river Vaitarni, are awaiting rebirth. How will they come back if she doesn't conceive?' His logic was simple. 'Moreover, what harm would a little bit of chanting and *baba's* antics do? We have been running from pillar to post for treatment for a long time, but to no avail.'

The woman looked indifferent. She was just a medium in the 'greater plan of things'. Years of subjugation had probably left her without a voice.

A long queue was piling outside. In a male dominated society, if a couple doesn't have a child, the problem is invariably attributed to the wife. A large number of women queue up outside infertility clinics, keen to shrug off the stigma of being 'barren' – a word people cruelly thrust upon them. Every cycle starts with hope, but by the end of month, it fades away. The long treatments, the cost crunch, and the frustration each month, takes its toll on the psyche and sees many dropouts.

We were surprised to see Shyama walk inside our room. Once, Shyama, too, had waited patiently outside this room. In her world, it was the duty of a woman to become a mother. She had been married for more than ten years, yet God had deprived her, and she had wallowed in self-pity. Stray rumours about her husband remarrying had reached her and inflamed her further. He loved her, but how long would he remain unwavering? A pair of blocked tubes had quashed her dreams of motherhood, forever. The only reprieve now was either a test tube baby, or IVF, but it was economically more feasible for her husband to remarry than indulge her fancy whims of maternity. Such a medical extravaganza was definitely out of bounds for her.

However, today she looked radiant and seemed to have gained a little weight. She could hardly contain herself and broke the news of her pregnancy proudly.

So she had finally got her IVF done, I asked.

'It was no IVF centre but our guru ji who did the miracle,' she told us smugly. 'I was desperate enough to try anything. He treated me with herbs which were neither expensive nor time-consuming, and I got pregnant within a few months. Just a day back, they tested me positive for pregnancy.'

Her guruji had ascended to the level of a living God for her. It was diplomatic to ignore the silent accusation in her eyes. 'A pair of blocked tubes' mocked us. If only God didn't make us look foolish, at times.

Another woman Leena's incredulous, 'I am pregnant!' still echoed in this clinic. For someone with one tube removed because of an ectopic (tubal) pregnancy and the other blocked pathologically, it was indeed a revelation. Five years back, faced with this major roadblock, she took to in vitro fertilization and was blessed with twin girls. Understandably, she never bothered about contraception after that. It was a shock when she missed her periods and turned out to be pregnant. She didn't want more children, yet was filled with unbridled joy. In her own words, she had lived a curse for far too long, and felt complete now. Strange was this feminine psyche, and strange was this phenomenon called motherhood.

Shyama elaborated how she was still in a very early stage of pregnancy, but all the distressing symptoms were already beginning to appear. She kept vomiting and felt weak all day.

Apart from simple reassurances and some medicines, there was not much we could offer. She was supposed to undergo some tests and an ultrasound a few weeks later. Shyama nodded and left.

She dropped in again, after nearly two months. Apart from having put on some more weight and a glow on her face, she had hardly any visible signs of pregnancy, which was nothing unusual as she was barely three months pregnant. She had brought some blood test reports which were normal, but there was no ultrasound report.

'Guruji has told us not to get it done as that can harm the baby. My mother is also against doing it. I have been getting regular check-ups done at the *ashram* (residence of a spiritual guru), and having medicines in the form of some powder.' She hesitated a little before admitting, 'I still trust this place so, against the advice of my family, I have come here.'

The importance of ultrasound notwithstanding, there was no means to force her. So we just advised and let go.

This guruji's magic potion remained a mystery. In all humility, we were ready to accept our deficiencies. Strangely, Shyama never told us the name of the guruji. Maybe it was a carefully guarded secret. Days passed by, but Shyama didn't show up again.

The daily routine sometimes threatens to become monotonous, but a controversy helps to break through the boredom. Lately, the city was abuzz with the news of the sensational arrest of a *baba*. It had caught people's fancy, and was all over the television and newspapers. With a list of bizarre activities to his credit, he sure was a prized catch for the police. People were shocked, as the man who they had once held in such high esteem – almost at par with God – was actually a mere criminal. He had succeeded in amassing a huge wealth, and was involved in offences as grave as drug trafficking and prostitution. There were reports of many frauds and scams, too. The nation watched, shocked, as once again a guru had brought shame to a nation known for its spiritual leaders. His properties had been sealed, yet it was surprising to see blind supporters protesting against his arrest and vouching for his innocence. With good connections and some well-known figures as his followers, he would have been out of jail if not for media pressure.

However, even a sensational news gets forgotten once you step into a hospital. Here, the only news that thrives is that which pertains to a patient. I entered the labour room and was greeted by a much rattled resident doctor.

'A labouring patient has just been admitted. Her abdomen is hugely distended and she was writhing in pain. I simply can't localize the baby's heartbeat.'

I was surprised to see our old patient Shyama, who had conceived with so much difficulty. Now nine months pregnant, she was lying there with labour pains. She could perceive the baby's movements well, till she started having pains about two hours back. I had not quite expected her to turn up at our hospital for delivery. Her whole abdomen was indeed very tight and bloated, making any examination difficult. As expected, there were hardly any blood tests done, apart from the ones we had done in the early stages of the pregnancy. And of course, the ultrasounds were pointedly absent. There were no papers from the place where she was getting her 'check-ups' done. Hoping that it was nothing serious, I sent her for a quick ultrasound, disregarding the protests by her attendants.

The ultrasound machine seemed to be in a mood to play gimmicks on us. All we could see on the trustworthy screen were bloated loops of gut. There was no trace of any baby inside. The uterus lay pushed to its virginal position, down into the pelvis hardly more than a few centimetres. Not wanting to believe what we were seeing, we restarted the machines but to no avail. Still not convinced, an experienced sonologist was called in.

A look at the patient, and he jibed, 'All you need to deliver is the gas, that's all!'

We were forced to acknowledge that in front of us, supposedly in labour, lay a patient of pseudocyesis, or phantom pregnancy. Many of us had never seen such a patient; only read about them in our medical textbooks.

It was almost surreal. Her obsession to have a child had reached disastrous dimensions. The supreme mind forced her to fake a pregnancy, and under stress, the periods stopped. The delusional woman even exaggerated acidity to pregnancy vomiting, and perceived bowel movements to a baby's movement inside the womb. Even those powdery medicines might have faked many symptoms of pregnancy. Thanks to the availability of ultrasound machines, these phantom pregnancies were detected early. The quack knew this psychology only too well, and indulged Shyama's fantasies. Or perhaps, it was her own subconscious mind that stopped her from getting an ultrasound. The 'pregnancy' progressed normally, and she landed up with labour pains which were actually intestinal colics. The highly imaginative power of the brain creates so many illusions and so many delusions!

The uphill task of breaking the news to Shyama and her relatives now loomed large. As expected, the patient went hysterical and her parents aggressive. A string of charges, from having botched up the case, to being vengeful and having a questionable intent, were thrown at our face. In all the hysteria, they let slip something interesting, too.

'If only our guruji was not in jail, and his place not sealed! Just a week back, guruji had himself checked and said that the baby was doing fine. He had even predicted that she would go into labour and be blessed with a baby boy. He had warned us from going anywhere else. Maybe it is that disgusting ultrasound machine that ate up the baby,' they wailed. The truth was slowly dawning on us.

Shyama and her family finally gave in to weeping inconsolably, mourning the loss of their precious baby. Somebody needed to talk some sense into them.

'It can be easily proven by medical evidence, that Shyama had never been pregnant. Unfortunately, the onus is on to you for being part of a carefully-hatched conspiracy, or probably being hand in glove with a much notorious and proclaimed offender.'

They panicked.

'Shyama's condition is a result of a psychological disorder that would need good counselling. But before that, she needs acceptance and family support.'

They were finally forced to accept that their 'higher-than-God' guruji had taken them for a ride.

Probably, Shyama needed some kind of shock to get out of this manipulative set-up. The truth was sinking in, and she gradually became less agitated. The accusations had stopped, and the relatives were now anxious about her. As our senior radiologist had suggested, we just needed to release all the gas held in her abdomen, and give her some strong analgesic to relieve her pain. She would see the psychiatrist tomorrow. However, before that, she needed some time to wear off the strain of her 'pregnancy'. She had lost a 'baby'. Her flight of fancy was pregnant with deceit and had consumed her fuels. She would drift for some time before she could become grounded again.

Finally, it was time for those on graveyard shifts to retire. Back home on the television, an excited reporter was gloating over the channel's latest breaking news. Fresh rounds of charges were made. A distraught mother was seen accusing the *baba* of stealing her newborn baby. She had delivered few days back, and had seen one of his aides, now in custody, behaving suspiciously in her ward. She had recognized him on television. The crowd went hoarse insisting for a CBI enquiry. The *baba* was shedding tears, and cried conspiracy.

With a knowing smile, I switched off the set. I was exhausted and let the darkness of the night engulf me. I took refuge in a world which was dark, yet free from the vices of a sinister mind. A world where a mind could live a dream, and not weave a nightmare to wake up to…

Yes, finally I went to sleep…

19
THE PLANNER

"Beyond the deeds of past,
the struggle and strife!
Future shrieked and cried.
As love laboured and sighed,
life opened its beautiful eyes.
Oh yes! The baby had arrived… "
(From my poem *Love's Labour,* published in the book *Dewdrops…*
a journey begins)

'But we never planned it!'

She had said that many times by now, but I had heard it the first time. The stage for planning was over, but at least, she was married. I kept hearing this from those who had yet to plan their wedding…

There has been tremendous advancement in medicine, but how people twist it to suit their way! Look at this woman. Faced with something which wouldn't have happened if she had really planned, she was desperate to be rid of it. Six months down the line, she would be back in the hospital, desperate to be pregnant again. It was strange that we didn't want to leave anything to God anymore.

'Man proposes, God disposes.' Ouch, did He say that? No, I guess I was the one who spoke aloud.

She pretended she had not heard it. They had already planned a trip to Europe. The tickets had been paid for, and hotels booked.

But a pregnancy was supposed to be more precious than a Europe trip!

But of course, the tickets were non-refundable. It was cheaper to 'refund' a pregnancy.

I knew when I had been cornered, and I knew when I had met a determined couple. If I didn't do it, they would move to the next doctor. After all, it was their right. The little, unborn baby, of course didn't even have the 'right to life'! In a fast-growing, overpopulous country like ours, we can't afford to debate this highly inflammatory topic, so it was better to let it go.

My next patient had a different agenda – a *mahurat* (auspicious time frame) delivery. Our most vicious rivals – the punditji or the family astrologer – were the ones most jealous of our 'next-to-God' status. This was their redemption time.

'Our punditji says that the most auspicious time for delivery is from twelve midnight till 1.30 am in the morning.'

The bait was thrown. Punditji was rubbing his hands in glee. We had these spats with the pundits so many times, yet they never gave up.

'How can I do a planned caesarean at midnight?'

'Not a caesarean, ma'am! I want a normal delivery.'

If she thought she was being generous, she should have looked into my furious eyes. Thankfully, she was too engrossed in her planning.

'Listen, how on earth can anyone promise you a normal delivery at a predetermined time? We can't give you labour pains with a preset alarm! I am not God, for God's sake!'

'Oh no ma'am, *aap to hamare liye bhagwan ho* (you are God for us)!'

And there she went! If ever there was an emotional blackmail of the worst degree, this was it. It always had the undesired effect and sent me through the roof. Why did she go to the punditji, when God and his 'standby' were both here?

Fuming, I went on to try making her realize the stupidity of what she was asking for. However, it fell on deaf ears.

'My in-laws trust this punditji a lot. He says that after 2 am, there will be bad *nakshatras* (alignment of heavenly bodies). It will be an inauspicious time after that.'

It was checkmate. Punditji was grinning ear to ear.

'Listen, please go and talk to him again. Let him suggest another time, preferably in the morning hours, and ask for a broader interval. Or else, you can have a caesarean.' That, too, was difficult, though more feasible.

Sometime back, a patient wanted a normal delivery on a Sunday, between twelve in the afternoon and 2 pm. She had got admitted on her own, without even consulting me. There was absolutely no emergency, and I didn't like her high-handedness. Sadly, she didn't like mine either, and delivered in the hospital at the next corner – a fact I didn't quite relish.

So, there was no point in being rudely dismissive. The patient was almighty. We had to bow down to her supreme command, and make a last minute landing in the operation theatre. We would be mocked by other doctors, especially those whose surgeries would be delayed for the *mahurat* delivery. But what choice did we really have?.

There was nothing new about these slanging matches with the pundits. Sometimes I felt they just relished our discomfiture. Ultimately, we would negotiate a better time. He would act magnanimous and grant me my wish. It was easy to manage a few minutes here and there in the theatre, but beyond that, it became difficult to manipulate. Maybe, the Smart Guy above enjoyed the spectacle that we made, trespassing his boundaries all the time. As it is, the 'Indian baby boom' would have strained him a lot and kept him busy, day and night...

If only we had some surprises in our kitty! Somehow, in the fast-paced lives that we lead, we totally missed out on them. On an impulse, I stopped at the bakery shop and picked up some cakes and goodies. My children would love the little surprise. These days, even friends never came uninformed any more, and parties had to be arranged well in advance. Memories from my now-distant childhood brought a strange longing in my heart and lit up my face with a reminiscent smile. That day, as I went to bed, I fervently wished God would spring some lovely surprise, and spice up this strangely predictable life that I was leading.

Mrs Sita Ramamurthy was a 50-year-old woman. Her family had settled in South Africa for three generations now. She was a South African at heart. Yet, she always wanted to visit this country her grandmother had often dreamily talked about. She had gotten married to Mr R Ramamurthy, another South African, whose family, like hers, had been settled in South Africa for generations. They had been planning to come to India for a long time, but somehow, the dream had kept eluding them till now. Their children had grown up, with the elder son now about 25 years old. She pampered them a lot like a typical Indian mom, yet they were as independent as their South African friends. She knew that they would now be able to manage on their own.

The 'rendezvous with India', as Mrs Ramamurthy called it, started as she waited excitedly to board the Air India flight at Johannesburg. She couldn't help feeling a slight heaviness in her abdomen. Maybe, it was the excitement of the last few days catching up. She had been trying her hand at a lot of Indian curries. Her tummy was not so used to the hot spices, but they always delighted her kids and she, too, secretly relished them. Now, there was gas and acidity that was bloating her abdomen. She must learn to be careful in India, too, she reminded herself sternly. Not realizing that she had laughed out loud, she saw her husband looking at her affectionately.

'Your excitement has brought a glow to your face. You have definitely started looking more beautiful.'

She blushed.

'You have put on more weight, too,' he chided gently.

This time she didn't mind being reminded about the extra inches on her forever-expanding waistline. Nothing could contain her happiness and it had spilled over to her face.

It was a long journey and Mrs Ramamurthy could hardly sleep. Her bowels kept moving all the time, and she kept shifting to ease off the pressure. Strangely, it made her breathless, too. If she was honest, she was getting that for quite a long time now. But then, she attributed it to the menopause she had had a year back. Her friend had once told her that such symptoms do happen and gradually settle down.

The changing phases of life! Maybe she should have seen her gynaecologist. Lines of worry appeared on her forehead, before she brushed them away. She would look at the Taj Mahal; the historically mystifying Delhi; and Chandni Chowk, where her grandparents had lived. The Paranthe Wali Gali kicked at her belly in anticipation. She had so much to look forward to. Smoothing out her furrows, she went to sleep.

She opened her eyes to her 'Midsummer Indian dream' as the plane landed at New Delhi. She was feeling better. Good that she hadn't worried her husband unnecessarily. She knew that he too was excited about the trip and looked forward to rediscovering his roots. They looked in awe at the Indian airport. It spoke richly of the splendour that was so ethnically Indian. It took almost an hour for them to complete the formalities.

Strangely, she felt a reluctance to walk and was forced to sit down. It was as if she was having cramps, and she had to rush to the washroom, twice. She was sure that she had upset her tummy. Her husband was now getting worried. They were met at the airport by their tour operator. He would be their guide for the next few days.

'I hope they have good hospitals in Delhi,' Mr Ramamurthy gently enquired, as he watched his wife clutching her abdomen in pain. The tour operator assured them, and gave her a painkiller he was carrying with himself. They thanked him for his kind gesture.

The journey to the hotel was fast enough, considering all that they had heard about the messy traffic in Delhi. They had barely checked into their room when Mrs Ramamurthy started doubling up in pain. The pressure in her lower abdomen was getting unbearable. A vague suspicion was forming in her head. There was a multi-specialty hospital that boasted of services at par with international standards hardly half a kilometre from their hotel, and the tour operator rushed them there.

I was seeing a patient who had been brought to the emergency, when a loud cry from the casualty medical officer rushed me to his side. Astonished by what I was seeing, I debated if we had enough time. However, taking my chances, I shifted her to the minor operation theatre in the casualty. We could be more comfortable there and have better privacy. There were instructions shouted left, right, and centre. She had been barely shifted to the trolley, that much to the astonishment of the surprised parents, we delivered a crying, healthy baby boy, anxious to be out on the Indian soil. I was thankful that somebody had remembered to call the paediatrician. We all rushed to congratulate the couple, but they gaped at us, reeling in shock. Shaking her head, the patient flopped down on the bed. Her husband watched bemused at the wonder that was wrapped up and given in his arms. And we listened disbelievingly, as they narrated their story of the baby's ignored existence.

'I thought it was menopause… No, I thought it was gas…!' the patient muttered incoherently.

'I thought she was getting fat…' her husband whispered, still in shock.

Well, wasn't it just yesterday that I was asking God for some nice little surprise! Even I had not thought that he would be listening to me, and act so fast. Maybe I should have asked for more!

We shifted them to a room where she could be more comfortable. They needed time to come to terms with reality. Leaving them with their bundle of surprise, I rushed off to the operation theatre.

The bad *nakshatras* were approaching and the baby had to be taken out fast. Punditji had conceded a little and suggested a morning time, but then there was no scope for normal delivery. With hardly any time to breathe, I couldn't be constrained any longer. Thankfully, she had agreed for a caesarean section. It was more important to deliver at a particular time, than the mode of delivery! I tried to look away from the glaring eyes of the surgeon whose case I had postponed. He would be calling me superstitious, but what could a poor doctor do when pitted against the stars? Anyway, the crash-landing in the theatre was less dramatic than the one we witnessed minutes before in the emergency!

The '*mahurat*' baby cried in jest, well ahead of the bad *nakshatras*. Leaving the beaming relatives fawning over it, I went to see the South African couple.

Mrs Ramamurthy was sleeping peacefully. Her husband, now out of shock, actually looked happy.

'Thank you, doctor, for this bundle of joy. You have started our second innings.'

'Thank you for being there in the nick of time. A little late, and the baby would have been born in the cab,' I could hardly hold back.

He laughed at that, relieved that it didn't actually happen.

'Have you broken the news to your kids?' I suddenly remembered his children back home.

'Of course.'

He showed me the images he had sent to them. His kids were over the moon.

'Awesome, dad. He is so cute,' I read the message, slowly.

They couldn't wait to see him and were planning to book their tickets to India. The family had finally discovered their Indian roots. I could bet that in India, grown-up children would have howled and died with shame, if blessed with a sibling at the age of twenty-five, and the parents humiliated and ridiculed by all. These people living abroad respected boundaries so much more, and gave each other breathing space. We had so much to learn from them. But yes, they should also learn a bit about *mahurats* from us.

I could imagine the Smart Guy winking at me.

'Thank you for the surprise. And don't worry! Next time when l ask you for something, I will be more specific,' I winked back at him...

20
THE BOND OF LOVE

"Beyond the veils of penury,
and the tales of misery,
Hope soared above the clouds,
Smiling at the bond of love…"

Balram was born as the son of Devki and Vasudeva, just like Krishna. However, to escape the fatal wrath of their uncle Kansa, he was transferred to the womb of Rohini, who was also Vasudeva's wife. She was childless and alone, while Vasudeva languished in captivity with his other wife. Rohini thus laid the roots of surrogacy for future generations to work on, and turn the myth to reality. What the Gods did in scriptures, ambitious human beings did in the present time with the aid of technology.

The concept of surrogacy is, hence, not new. It is a boon to the failing dreams of childless couples. Many such people flock to India because of the easy availability of surrogates at an astonishingly low cost. Braving attacks by activists and reeling under the stigma of exploiting poor women for money, India continues to bring a smile on the faces of couples who had lost hope. India understands the plight of infertile women more than the West, for here, it was not only a mental trauma but also a social travail. The practice of surrogacy thrives on the universal and very primitive need of people to survive and procreate.

Lifting the curse from an infertile woman, surrogacy saved her marriage. A husband didn't need to dump his wife and remarry, neither, in true Bollywood style, did a woman need to push her husband into the arms of any other woman, any longer.

However, we live in times of changing social patterns and moral values. Sometimes, people have hidden agendas. Surrogacy threatens to break many rules made by nature and imposed by culture. Thus, it gets marred with controversies. I remembered Deepa, whose baby I had delivered about five years back.

She had been referred to us by the IVF department when she was four months pregnant. I knew she was a surrogate mother. She had a 10-year-old son, and her husband had recently lost his job. They required money, as even the most bare essentials were becoming hard to afford. They decided to do this as the money was attractive. She had not asked for any favours for she felt that she was doing a 'job' and getting paid for it. I was always impressed by her straightforwardness. She didn't like saying that she had rented out her womb; rather she believed that somebody had borrowed her womb. Yet, that 'someone' remained conspicuous by his absence. Generally, we got to know about the biological parents, but here it was a mystery. Nobody was too forthcoming, and I didn't want to sound inquisitive. In the later months of pregnancy, Deepa developed high blood sugar, and had to be put on insulin. It was risky for the baby if the sugars went too high. She had to follow a strict diet and rigorous blood sugar testing. The daily insulin injections were also no less painful. I could see scabs from multiple punctures on her skin.

'So much strain, so much pain for somebody else's baby, Deepa?'

'So what? Don't you work hard, struggle hard for someone else's baby?' she replied tartly. She loved her job, just as I did. Deepa always put the ball in my court.

'If you have a caesarean delivery again, it'll make future deliveries more complicated,' I said.

However, she was not worried.

'I don't plan to have any more children for myself. I love this baby growing inside me. It is going to be with me only for nine months and I want to relish every moment. Right now, it's my baby and I will nurture it with love. So what if I am getting money in return?'

Her son and mother-in-law often came with her to listen to the baby's heartbeat.

'Isn't your family curious? Doesn't your son ask questions?'

'A child's world is different from ours. With time, he'll understand. After all, I am doing this for his better future.'

'Then came the day when we had to decide her date of delivery. The biological father wanted it two days later, on his own birthday. The couple was coming to meet me'. As I waited, I saw the IVF specialist usher in a couple inside my clinic. To my surprise, they were both foreigners. She introduced the father, who looked like he would be in his early thirties. The old woman sitting next to him was his mother.

So, where was the baby's mother? Before I could dwell much on this, another man, a foreigner again, entered our cabin.

'Sorry, doc, for being late! Hope the baby's doing fine? So, are we doing the caesarean two days later?' He sounded quite enthusiastic about the baby.

'Yes! Now you can look forward to celebrating your birthday with your baby,' I nodded, looking pointedly at the father.

The 'father' shook his head and pointed towards his friend who had just entered, 'Actually, doc, that's his birthday.'

So, he was the father! How could there be two fathers? I was going to voice that aloud when comprehension dawned. I slowly looked at both of them, then at his mother who had come to take care of the baby, and then at our IVF specialist. Her eyes confirmed my suspicion.

Deepa had a caesarean two days later, and the baby handed over to the proud fathers.

'I don't want to see the baby,' she declared, as she stared impassively. 'My role in his life is over.'

I understood her. Her job was not as easy as mine. The foreign couple was ecstatic. I didn't want to be judgemental. We live in a world pregnant with possibilities. If there was a will and an obvious way, then even God couldn't stand in the path. Science and technology had ensured that...

There was a reason I was remembering Deepa today. Another tryst with destiny had come to an end. However, the passengers were much different and they had each lived a unique story. Today, they waited to embark on separate paths.

I looked outside.

A woman stood quietly in a corner oblivious to all, watching intently the baby sleeping in her arms. This was a moment to be savoured – a parent beholding a blissfully sleeping infant. They all looked like angels in sleep. She had waited for this moment for so long. Fate had tormented her. God had taken a long time to be kind.

Three years back, she had entered the hospital in severe pain. Pushing open the door of the labour ward and thumping her abdomen with both her hands, Nikita had wailed and shouted for help. She was wheeled inside; a desperate woman who was almost hysterical, despite assurances. Was it pain, or was she fighting the demons of an unforgiving past?

'Save my baby. It will die!' she moaned desperately.

'Hey, don't be so negative! You are in a hospital now. You will be fine.'

'You don't understand! It's like that every time! They come out well, but die soon after birth for no apparent reason. I have lost two babies like this before. It will happen again!'

Her eyes reflected her panic, and her hands squeezed her tummy as bouts of agony gripped her. She was laid on the hospital bed. The baby's heartbeat was fine, but her abdomen, tense. After her last pregnancy, she had had a fibroid removal done. Her womb, scarred by the previous surgery, was probably not being able to tolerate the added stress of labour pains. It had already been weakened and stretched beyond limits by the present pregnancy. We decided to take her up for surgery quickly. As she was being shifted, the baby's heartbeat shifted its position upwards, causing us to worry.

On opening her up, our fears were confirmed when we saw the baby lying motionless in the abdomen, outside a badly torn uterus. It had thrown the baby out of the womb, bloodless and severing all connections. Life had deserted the baby and the rescue team was late by just a few minutes. To make matters worse, her uterus was split in two parts, like two halves of a fruit, and bleeding profusely. It could not be salvaged and had to be removed. She stayed in the ICU for two days. No one told her anything, yet, strangely, she knew and accepted her fate. She had tried thrice, yet destiny had so inhumanely snatched her moment of happiness every single time, with appalling shrewdness. How would she trust it anymore? She had been tense throughout the entire pregnancy, as if anticipating this very moment. She finally had her worst fears confirmed.

Her husband was broken, yet he was her pillar of support. 'We plan to settle abroad now, and we'll think of adoption later, if Nikita is still willing. The desire for a baby had consumed us, but we need to look at a life with different prospects, now. I don't want to keep fighting for something fate has not willed for us.' His resigned tone belied his composure.

Two years later, I again saw her outside the infertility clinic. Surrogacy was her only option to have a biological child, and they were tempted to try once. She was living abroad. The cost of treatment there was beyond her, and she had come back to her motherland. Everything here was cheap. Even a womb could be rented at astoundingly low figures, as the cost of survival for some people was still very high.

She was back in the hospital. The goal was the same, but the road was different. She needed someone suitable who could carry her dream for nine months, nurture it with the love of a mother, and yet cut the bond at birth and deliver it safely in her arms. A baby at a cost! And she wanted someone who would take the cost and deliver her the baby.

Radha had been living a life of misery. Married off by her poor parents at a young age of eighteen, she never had the time to study properly. Her husband worked in a garment shop. They struggled to make their ends meet. Their ignorance saw them giving birth to two daughters in quick succession. Things were getting expensive and they, frustrated. Her husband fell in bad company and started drinking. That further gnawed into the crumbling walls of her home, and consumed whatever money was left. They now fought daily, and gradually her marriage turned ugly and fragile. He became alcoholic and abusive, and one day, he beat her badly. Sick of him, she left home with her two daughters.

She had never known how to fend for herself and hardly knew any vocation other than doing housework. She started working as a maid and rented a room near her parents' house. Still, there was never enough food for all three of them. She could hardly think of sending her daughters to school. Her husband still came sometimes, just to fight with her and take away all the money she had. There were many nights when they had to sleep on empty stomachs. In her own words, she kept a stick with her. When her children cried, she tried to make them sleep. If they didn't, she gave them water. If they still didn't, she hit them, and the poor kids along with their helpless mother, cried themselves to sleep. The kindness of the people she worked with made some days happy, yet the future of her daughters seemed vague with such a meagre income.

One day, Radha was working when she heard her mistress talking to her friend about infertility centres looking out for surrogates. They were talking about a good amount of money given by these places to those who agreed to rent their womb. Radha was interested, and asked for details. Her mistress looked surprised, but she was kind and knew her circumstances well. She gave her the address and the phone number. Radha couldn't stop thinking about it. It was a little bizarre and unheard of, yet it tempted her with possibilities. She didn't have many people to discuss with, but as she lay at night and looked at the innocent faces of her sleeping daughters, it suddenly looked much viable.

A week later, nervous to the core, she was sitting inside the surrogacy clinic. They were nice people and spoke to her kindly. Everything was explained to her in details. They counselled her, and she met a lawyer who told her about her rights and duties as well. She had to be fit to undergo the whole procedure. That meant a whole lot of tests. They assured her of her safety, and offered her an attractive package, something she had never dreamt of earning in her life.

Yet, she came back home, apprehensive. She was scared that people would talk about her. How would she justify herself to her daughters? And what would happen if something went wrong with her? She was worried about the girls.

She decided to meet her husband. His consent was mandatory before things moved any further. Moreover, she didn't want him casting aspersions on her character, if she got pregnant. So next day, she went to see him at his place. With hardly any preamble, she told him about her plan. He listened to her and, to her disbelief, agreed to what she proposed. Maybe it was the money that lured him, but suddenly, he was all attentive. He promised to go along with her. On her way back, Radha realised the importance of money. She felt strangely empowered. For the first time, her husband believed she was worthy enough. It filled her with confidence and pride. It had not been easy living alone. She remembered her early days of marriage when they were not rich, but not exactly unhappy, either. Maybe, he was regretting, too. The more she thought about it, the more feasible it seemed. The promise of a secure future beckoned her and after a long time, she slept peacefully that night.

The next few days went in a flurry of tests. She was young and healthy, and it worked in her favour. She was chosen to be a surrogate mother to the baby of Nikita and her husband Sahil.

Nikita and Sahil had their own reasons to be apprehensive. Their tryst with destiny had not exactly been kind. They didn't want fate to dupe them again, and were worried about the intentions of the surrogate mother. All legalities were in place, but she might just run away with their baby as well as the money. It would get messy, and they didn't want to fight dirty in the Indian courts. The infertility centre assured them. They needed to trust and respect their surrogate. Radha could hardly fend for her two children; she definitely didn't want to be saddled with any more. She understood all that was required of her. Her priority was to get rid of her penury, more than anything else.

Soon, Radha's journey began. She was pregnant with their baby. The cost of her treatment was taken care of. She was well provided for so that she could eat, and her family didn't have to sleep hungry. She managed to put her daughters in a trust school with the help of the hospital. Her husband, who was still surprised by the turn of events, started living with her.

Radha was raising a life; how could she possibly not care for it? It was bliss to feel the baby moving inside her. It filled her with pure maternal love. But this was a job she was doing. She reminded herself that when she cleaned somebody's home, she couldn't live in it, and neither could she eat the food that she cooked in their houses. Radha wanted to do her job well, and didn't want to disappoint those who were promising her a better life.

With time, Nikita and Sahil learned to accept Radha. They looked forward to the progress card and ultrasound images the hospital sent them. With every passing day, Nikita's happiness grew along with a nagging fear. It was God she feared above everything else. How could she trust him again? However, the doctors soothed her. Radha had no pre-existing problems. There was no point being pessimistic.

Radha didn't hide the nature of her pregnancy from anyone. Nobody spoke anything in front of her, and she was not bothered by what others said behind her back. Life was happy and relaxed for the first time. Her husband was a changed and sincere person now. Probably, he looked forward to a comfortable life as well.

Soon the day came when both the women were going to bear the fruit of their labour. Radha gave to Nikita what even the Gods had denied her. She was too astounded to speak and looked at the baby in wonder. Nikita and Sahil celebrated their little bundle of joy, while Radha recovered in the post-operative ward, suffering pain, as her job tenure ended. She had earned money, but the tears of happiness on the face of the couple were no less of a reward. It filled her with purpose. The couples understood each other, for both of them had done this for their children. She didn't know the legalities, or understand what the moral brigades were protesting against. This had given her happiness, and a secure life she had never dreamt of earlier. Given a chance, she might do it again. A new source of employment had been generated. She didn't want to go back to the hell of poverty.

Sahil and Nikita were leaving the country tomorrow. They had come to meet Radha, who was there for her post-natal check-up. They hugged each other. Nikita had brought gifts for Radha and her girls. They clicked pictures with the woman who had given them the gift of life. She was more than God to them. They promised to send her snaps of the baby as it grew up. Radha would miss the little baby, and the couple who had given her a new identity, and her family, a new lease of life. In her own way, the surrogate mother would forever be in debt to the couple.

The umbilical cord may have been cut, but they were now bound forever. A 'bond of love' would always keep them together.

21
AN UNTAMED JUNGLE

"Each day,
a different story
hidden in the seams,
slowly unfolds.
Each day,
a different folly
hidden in dubious plots,
lies untold…"

'I can't!'

I looked back at the anxious eyes of the woman who was refusing to lie down on the examination table. I had tried to coax her into lying down so many times, yet she sprang up every time I moved towards her.

'I won't hurt you. It's just a routine check-up,' I tried to assure her once again.

She was a 40-year-old woman, married for the last fifteen years. I had just met her husband, a handsome army officer, who was quite worried about the lower abdomen pains she kept having off and on.

'I can't help it.' She looked at me tearfully. Beads of sweat were waiting to trickle down her forehead. Her clenched limbs, tightly clasped together, conveyed a fear blown out of proportion. I didn't want to lose my patience.

'You have been married for fifteen years and have a son, too!'

'Actually, he is adopted. I could never really...' her voice trailed off as she looked at me miserably.

Comprehension was dawning on me, slowly. 'It's all right. You can come down. Next time, I will take you under anaesthesia even for a check-up.' I tried to laugh.

She smiled back thankfully. Her relief on getting down the table was almost palpable.

'Well, you get an ultrasound done. That can tell us quiet a lot of things. However, even that can't take the place of a direct examination.'

'I am sorry. I have never been able to overcome this fear that has made my life miserable. My husband – you know – we never actually had any physical relation.'

I could already make that out, but didn't want to prod much. I simply nodded sympathetically.

'You must have taken professional help.'

'Initially, we thought it was just something like early, marriage jitters. I got married quiet young. But as days passed, we realised that this almost pathological, a morbid fear. I used to feel so awful that, at times, I even thought of taking my life. It was then that we decided to take professional help. We consulted a psychiatrist. I had it all – sessions of counselling, medicines, and even an examination under anaesthesia. But nothing really helped. I was diagnosed as suffering from an intractable vaginismus. In the end, we decided to put an end to all suffering, and I quit trying.'

'Your husband?' It was out before I could stop myself.

'He never made any demands on me. He believed me when I said I loved him. I even offered to divorce him but he would not hear of it. Maybe he understood the demons that wracked me, and accepted me just as I am. He loves me too much to destroy me.'

It sounded too good to be true, but I kept that to myself. She was lucky to have such a husband.

'Indeed, I am lucky. He is such a darling,' she said happily, as if she could read my mind.

A few minutes later, the 'darling' walked into my chamber and affectionately put his arms around her. Honestly, I didn't know such men existed. The cynic in me threatened to rise and taunt once again, but I clamped it down. I should stop judging people, and mind my own business. That something called 'love', I mused.

No sooner had she left that our nurse Chanda came rushing towards me. She blurted out excitedly, 'Madam, that patient has brought her neighbour to the hospital today, all alone. She asked me to tell you that. You remember, the one whose husband didn't let her talk, or come to the hospital on her own? The one you had scolded?'

I scolded quite a few, I said, grinning. But I remembered the one she was talking about.

I had called her an indirect patient because everything about her came indirectly, through her know-it-all husband. You ask her something and she would look at him. The superior male mentality! The moment she opened her mouth, he would promptly answer as if not trusting her to be right. Maybe, he didn't credit her with any intelligence. Be it the number of children she had or her mode of delivery, he knew better. It actually became ludicrous when we came to her menstrual history. She started to speak, but then looked at him for confirmation. Reveling in his knowledge, he interrupted her and went on all about her dates and her periodicity in absurd detail. He was getting on my nerves. I generally didn't let gentlemen of this kind stay in the room, but some insistent ones refused to go. I had to interrupt him a bit too forcefully, 'Can she speak?'

'Madam, *isko kuch samajh nahi aata. Bahut bholi hai bechari.* (Madam, she doesn't understand anything. She is very innocent.) She gets scared easily.' He added generously, '*Batao, batao, tum theek se batao sub kuch.* (Go on, say everything properly.)'

The poor woman stammered, too conscious to speak in his presence.

I always wondered how such women brought up their kids. Or maybe, the husbands interfered in this, too.

'Of course not, madam. But, *kya karein* (what to do)? She has no confidence.'

I didn't realise that I had spoken out aloud. And he didn't realise he was insulting her.

'Maybe this has happened because you don't allow her to speak at all.'

He was quick to deny that.

'If a woman is not confident, it's either her parents' or her husband's fault.'

That made him happier. He could now shift the blame. New punching bags – her parents! Well, he had to move out and the woman had to talk. However, by the time that happened, she was almost in tears. She looked shamefaced, but accepted that he never let her talk much.

'But did he ever stop you from fighting with your neighbours or your mother-in-law?'

That made her laugh a little, but she shook her head in the negative. She had to own some responsibility.

This was her second pregnancy and she was already five months pregnant. Her husband didn't have time to bring her to the hospital. They lived in the capital city of the country, yet the woman could not come for a check-up alone. I have never understood this dependency women had on their husbands.

I was quiet for some time before I said, 'If a woman cannot travel alone, then even I should not come to the hospital alone. Maybe, next time you should go to a male doctor.'

'It's not like that. You are a doctor, and I, a housewife.'

She looked after a whole family – the family builder! Yet she believed that she couldn't do it! How would anyone respect her, if she remained buried in her husband's shadows?

Shrugging, I went on to write down her prescription and then explained in detail the medicines she had to take. She listened, but then requested me to repeat everything to her husband.

Why should I do that, I asked.

'Well, actually he wouldn't believe me.'

I refused and she walked out reluctantly. Five minutes later, the gentleman entered with my prescription in his hand. He asked to be explained.

'But I have already explained!'

'She hasn't understood properly.'

I could bet that he had not even asked her.

'Oh! Is she less intelligent, or are you wiser?'

'*Arre nahi, ma'am. Woh gaon ki hai na.* (Oh no, ma'am. She has come from a village.)'

It was an excuse, not a fact. Were villagers dumb people?

I patiently asked her to come inside and explain everything. Much to his annoyance, she repeated everything that I had advised, to perfection.

It was just his constant domination that had made her underconfident, and nothing else.

'Next time, let her come alone if you are busy,' I said to his retreating back. Nothing wrong in gloating a little.

She turned and passed me a shy smile...

I smiled to myself as I came back to the present. It felt good to see women respecting and rediscovering themselves.

There was somebody else waiting to see me today. He had crossed miles to be here, with his wife. These were days of medical tourism and India, with her affordable and quality healthcare, was fast becoming a hotspot for patients from all over the world, especially the Third World countries. An African girl asked me if she could come inside. It was a major relief that she could converse in English, as with the interpreters, one had to solely trust their wisdom.

She sat next to me, obliquely, and an old man with a black stick walked inside. I was surprised to know that he was her husband; she could have easily passed off as his daughter. There was an unmistakable air of authority around him.

An intractable infection had brought the girl to India. She turned slightly, and I was startled by the sound of a baby crying. A wrap had been turned into a sling, and a small baby was sleeping comfortably on her back, inside it. She had two more kids. Her husband moved out to make the baby quiet, using the black stick to guide himself.

His wife saw my eyes following him, and told me quietly, 'He has a bad vision.'

I couldn't help noticing that she looked very young.

'I am twenty-six and he is seventy-three,' she told me bitterly.

'Oh!' I said. 'You must have married really young.'

'I was fourteen when I got married. Being an orphan at the mercy of my relatives, I had no choice.'

'Does he have more wives?'

'We are four of us,' she stated as a matter of fact.

He must be having grandchildren her age!

She was suffering from a bad infection, probably a sexually-transmitted one. I found an infected loop that needed to be removed. Loops were intrauterine devices for preventing pregnancies. However, the mere mention of the loop scared her immensely.

'Please do not to tell him anything about it,' she pleaded with me. 'I got it inserted much against his wishes. He had asked me to remove it.'

Obviously she had not.

'I don't want more kids and can't trust him. He is the one infecting all the wives, yet refuses to even see a doctor. He is such an obstinate guy. Just yesterday, the eye specialist said that his vision could not be improved much. Rather than accepting that, he got extremely agitated. I asked him to be patient, but he just lost it.'

There were ugly marks on her wrist. Worse, it had all happened in the safe boundaries of a hospital.

'I don't know how he will react if he discovers this secret that lies buried inside me. He's never the one to take defiance easily.'

It was tough to hide something which could easily be seen on an ultrasound, but one could try to be a little diplomatic. I called him inside.

'The loop has not been taken out properly. An ultrasound can easily confirm that.'

He looked thoughtful but nodded his head.

Getting confident, I continued, 'The loop may be the culprit causing so much infection. But both the partners need to be checked and treated, otherwise even you might get afflicted.' He agreed readily.

She thanked me silently, and with the baby once again slung on her back, they both left, promising to come back with the reports.

Phew! So it was not only India. Women from other countries, too, suffered from such rampant abuse.

I saw them again a few days later, with the reports. Thankfully, she had responded to the antibiotics and I removed the offending loop. I, once again, requested the husband to keep a distance from her or he would be in serious trouble. There was not much I could do beyond that. He had still not gotten himself tested, nor had he started any treatment. His larger-than-life male ego prevented him from getting a check-up done. He appeared to be somewhat of a powerful, old lord of his country. But she was still so young!

'How long would you put up with his atrocities?'

'I have a sister who lives in America. She can help me, but every time I think of leaving him, my children pull me back. What if I fail look after them, alone? Should I deprive them of their rich legacy? I can't be so selfish.'

I had no answers. Her grim future stared back at me.

Pity is a sobering expression, and it stayed in my mind long after she had left. Women in India were not alone. A poor woman at the mercy of a rich man; the story repeated itself beyond boundaries and beyond time zones. Once again, poverty and illiteracy were the culprits, and women, the vulnerable victims.

The mind is an untamed jungle, and might, a wild animal. The mighty would always dominate and the weak would fall prey, till the mind is bound by rules, and culture prevails. Hopefully, tomorrow would be another day...

22
THE TRANSFORMATION

"Neither a myth
nor a figment of imagination,
A daring truth
not a glaring fiction;
Something real stares at you
in silent condemnation..."

She was tired. It was an effort to keep her eyes open. She had been trying to sleep all through the day, but the persistent 'demands' kept her awake. The sleepless nights were taking their toll. It was such a pleasure to close her eyes. The darkness welcomed her. Just for a while, she could pretend that all this had not happened, and she was free. She inhaled deeply. The sound of a wailing baby intruded on her senses. She tried hard to push it away, but it kept coming close. It was now irritating her. She pressed her ears, and closed her eyes tightly. Damn it!

A new patient was being sent to the labour room. No, she wasn't in labour. She had already delivered. Readmitted in the post-natal ward with vague psychiatric symptoms, she was turning out to be an enigma to many. In the evening, to the horror of those present, she had tried to jump from the balcony of the post-natal ward which was on the sixth floor. It had been difficult to restrain her. With the absence of a psychiatric ward in the hospital, she was to be kept in the labour ward temporarily for close supervision. The strict enclosures ensured more safety.

As I watched with curiosity, a young woman with disheveled hair was wheeled inside the labour ward. She was allotted a bed near the nursing station so that the nurses could keep a vigil over her. As she turned, I recognised her with a shock. It was Noorin, our old patient. She had delivered nearly a month back. I looked at her with trepidation. The woman I once knew stood transformed, barely discernible.

She was put down, with difficulty, on her bed. I reached out to touch her pulse, and she recoiled.

'Noorin, *teri amma kaun hai* (who's your mother)?' she spoke irrelevantly, as if in a trance.

I asked her to lie down, but she seemed miles away from me, lost in her own world. She looked at me, but I could sense that she looked beyond me. It was creepy. Once again, I tried to examine her, and again she sprang up.

'Noorin, *teri amma kaun hai?*'

I struggled to comprehend what she was trying to say, but failed. She had almost killed her own baby. The dichotomy going on in her brain had wiped the beauty from her face, and she looked fierce. I was bewildered. Something was terribly wrong here. Her parents were looking after Noorin, and had brought her in. I had to talk to them. A celebrated physiology called childbirth, had turned into a regretful pathology. Was it a fallout of the stressful lives we led? Or was it indeed just the neurotransmitters and some wayward hormones that pregnancy wreaked havoc on? The graph of these emotionally vulnerable patients was rising. Was it a mere coincidence that, just a few days back, I had met a much distressed husband of another patient who was in deep crisis? As

I waited for Noorin's mother, I recalled meeting Arjun, who had come to my clinic, not really understanding what was happening to his once-happy world.

He had had a baby a month back. Since his wife Devrina got pregnant, his world had changed. He was paranoid about her diet and well-being. Looking forward to each visit, he could hardly contain his joy at the sound of the baby's heartbeat. If it was within his power, he would have an ultrasound every few days, just to peek in and say a quick hello to his baby. Devrina was not exactly a submissive person, but she never looked suffocated by his attention. His excitement carried on throughout the pregnancy, but towards the end he got jittery. He just couldn't allow her to undergo so much pain. His wife laughed it off and chose to have a normal delivery. It was hilarious to see everyone supporting the much-in-distress husband while his wife laboured reasonably well. If only we could give a good dose of anaesthesia to him as well.

A father was born that day in our labour room. Simply over the moon at the sight of his little princess, he spent most of his time looking after her. He couldn't even trust her with the grandparents. In the initial days when the baby was not feeding well, Devrina was asked to be patient and persistent in her efforts, but it was so difficult to contain the desperate father. His solutions were almost surreal and comical. Unable to get a leave of more than two weeks, he resigned from his job. He planned to work from home for the next few months till his daughter was settled. There were not many men who would leave their jobs to look after a newborn baby, even if they could afford it. Unlike others, he was rather happy to be a house husband and a 'nursing' father, while she rested and relaxed. At times, his attention bordered on obsession, but then, maybe we were a tiny bit jealous as we were not used to having such men around.

However, that day he sat quietly. He had come alone, without Devrina. I could make out that he was disturbed. His wife was not behaving like a typical mother. He was doing his best to help her, but she got irritated easily. He attributed it to lack of sleep, and willingly got up in the night to take care of the baby. At times, he was forced to give the baby top-up feeds, too, and yet she behaved oddly. Whenever the baby got up and started crying, she would complain; at times, mouthing expletives too. He had never heard these words from her, and was shocked. He tried to talk to her but she was strangely withdrawn. In spite of his assurances and ready support, it continued. A few days back, after its feeding session, the little baby continued to be cranky and refused to sleep. Arjun had just closed his eyes. Suddenly his eyes flew open when he saw an agitated Devrina scolding the baby and throwing him on the bed in frustration. Luckily he was there. The startled expression on the baby's face, as it flopped helplessly on the bed, haunted him for days. Devrina was equally tearful and was consumed by guilt, when confronted. She didn't appear to be in control of her actions. She clung to him and begged him not to leave her alone with the baby.

To make matters worse, she started suffering from a strange obsession. One day, while giving the baby a bath, a strange thought entered her mind: if the baby was left in the tub, would she drown?

It scared her, yet there was a strange fascination that kept her thinking about it. The next day she was gripped by another distressing thought: if she closed her hands around the baby's neck, would she strangulate? Would she actually die?

It was frightening, but the thought clung to her mind. She tried to shrug it off, but it refused to go. She even attempted to close her hands around its neck, and, as the baby choked, she withdrew her hands, horrified. She was ashamed, and scared to be near the baby. Damning thoughts now engulfed her and were taking away her peace of mind. She had laboured for this baby, so why was she now so full of such fatal thoughts? It filled her with dread, but she was helpless against the obsession that compelled her to think like this. She was getting reduced to a bundle of nerves. Like a fish caught in the net, she floundered, begging release.

Arjun's dream of a happy family lay shattered. At night, he was forced to sleep in-between them. Devrina insisted that he stayed around always, so that she wouldn't end up harming their baby. His world stood devastated and he was at a loss to comprehend her strange obsessions. He loved his wife, but their daughter needed unconditional love from her mother, too. Her fears had created an impossible gulf that he failed to bridge, despite all his efforts.

I could understand his distress as well as the bizarre behaviour of his wife. She was probably suffering from obsessive compulsive neurosis, which might be having an element of post-partum depression. It was not very uncommon, though very few people came forward to acknowledge it. Maybe it was the changing dynamics in her body, or the demands after delivery,but something had made her prone to depression. Her husband obviously found it difficult to accept the unexpected behaviour of his wife. It was nobody's fault, but she needed immediate medical attention. She had, at least, retained some semblance of logic, and had not yet developed frank psychosis. With his love and support, she could tide over this moment of crisis. The lines of worry on his face eased off slightly. He promised to come back with Devrina to see the psychiatrist soon.

It was uncanny that so soon after coming to know about Devrina, I would be meeting another patient who had lost control of that delicate balance that keeps our sanity intact. Maybe, God wanted me to accept our failures in unravelling the secrets that lay buried inside our grey matter.

The sound of footsteps coming near, broke my reverie. Somebody was walking purposely towards the windows. The dress looked vaguely familiar. She opened the windows and started struggling with the iron grills. Realization hit, and I rushed towards her. Was she attempting to jump from the window? Before I could reach her, the woman turned, frustrated by failed attempt. I was shocked to see Noorin, with a face which was totally devoid of any expression.

'My clothes! She is wearing my clothes, oh God!' the labour room nurse shrieked.

Before going on with their duties, the nurses used to change into their uniforms in the changing room. Noorin had quietly sneaked in there and worn one of the nurses' dress and heels. It was beyond anyone to question her, or understand the workings of a mind that had gone totally haywire. From the corner of my eye, I noticed the ward *bai* trying to cover her mouth to stifle a laugh. The stigma in the Indian society that ridiculed patients suffering from mental illness as 'crazy lunatics', came to my mind. They needed to be empathised with, not mocked. Mental illness was more frightening than a physical disease. The mind was an unexplored territory, and she was at war with her own mind. Sternly reprimanding the ward *bai*, I sent her to fetch Noorin's mother.

An anxious woman, who introduced herself as Noorin's mother, walked inside hesitatingly. Lines of worry were etched deep into her face. The celebration of childbearing was over, and a thick pall of gloom had descended over their family. On my gentle prodding, she wiped her teary eyes and narrated to me the events that had preceded their arrival at the hospital.

Noorin had always been their pride. An intelligent and hard-working girl, she had built a comfortable life for herself. She got married two years back, to Saurabh, who had been her batchmate and friend.

His parents were initially against this marriage and had problems with Noorin, but with time, things were settling down – or so they believed. She had met Noorin briefly in the seventh month of pregnancy, when she appeared a little strained. However, they were least prepared with what met their eyes, when she arrived at their doorstep a fortnight ago with the baby in her arms. She lacked the glow of new-found motherhood on her face. Rather, she behaved quite indifferently, and was accompanied by a husband who was probably unaware of the turmoil going inside her.

Since her pregnancy, Noorin hardly had anyone to look after her. Her husband was always busy, and took it for granted that whenever needed, his parents would step in. But how they bugged her! Their non-stop chatter and undue interference took away whatever little peace was left. Their demands on her grew along with the pregnancy. This strained her relations with her husband too.

Soon, the baby stopped growing. For someone who had always been successful, she was now failing, first with Saurabh, and now with her baby. She loved the baby, yet could not make it grow. Her dreams of a content and blissful life now seemed such a mirage.

The pregnancy dragged on with difficulty, till one day, she finally delivered. A thin and gaunt baby boy, who looked almost like an old man, whimpered in her arms. The long period of stress had famished the little one, and this showed in the wrinkles all over him. Somehow, he was always hungry and never stopped crying. When it was time for everyone to sleep, he would wake up. The days were equally bad. She was tired, and for all her efforts, the baby didn't even give a smile. With no help, she was on the verge of collapsing. Taking pity, her husband dropped her at her parents' house, and went back, relieved. However, sadly for her parents, their cheerful daughter had disappeared, and instead, they met an agitated woman in her place. The dark circles under her eyes, and her blanched face, made her look severe.

They tried to reach out to her many times, but she remained detached and impassive. They blamed it squarely on her in-laws, and completely failed to fathom the storm that was brewing in her mind, till they were rudely awakened.

One day, they woke up to the cry of her baby. In a fit of rage, Noorin had thrown him on the floor, and was looming over him, dangerously. They had never seen her in such a bad temper. Scared, her mother took the bruised baby in her arms. He, fortunately, had escaped unhurt, but since that day, they made it a point to not leave their daughter alone with the baby. They tried to reason out with her gently, but neither did Noorin bat an eyelid, nor did she show any remorse. Something was definitely wrong, but they didn't want to acknowledge the fact that their daughter was losing her sanity. The constant visits by relatives, and the customary celebrations that followed childbirth in an Indian household, further prevented them from coming to terms with the pathology that had crept in, uninvited, to their house.

The poor parents were still debating about how to talk to their son-in-law, when Noorin did the unthinkable. It was a quiet afternoon when Noorin's mother, tired after rocking the baby to sleep, decided to take a nap. She didn't know that Noorin was silently walking up the stairs. Her father was talking to his neighbour in front of their house. Suddenly, a loud noise made them turn their heads, and they saw Noorin land on a pile of sand in front of their house, with a loud thud. They rushed her to the hospital. Miraculously, she sustained only minor injuries probably because she had fallen over a heap of sand. It was sheer luck that her parents had locked the door to the second floor and she couldn't reach the top of the house.

Her mother's small body rocked, as she sobbed uncontrollably. If only they knew what had usurped her happiness. Noorin had become a slave to an unbending mind. It was always hard to accept a mental illness, especially following moments of jubilation like childbirth. She was living a paradox.

Noorin was showing definite symptoms of post-partum psychosis. I could do nothing other than console her mother. At least, we knew what plagued her. The psychiatrist was on the way, and so was Noorin's frightened husband.

So much goes on in the mysterious mind. Sensitive to the interplay of chemicals in the closed circuit of the brain, we are still far from unravelling what triggers a catastrophe.

I looked at Noorin as she slept peacefully under the influence of drugs. The nurses had finally managed to put her to bed. Praying silently that her mind would not wake up to the nightmare her life had turned into, I squeezed her mother's shoulders. It was time she went home to take care of Noorin's baby.

The path to recovery was tough, but not entirely impossible. Medicines didn't have the power of love and care. She would need every inch of their support to sail through this moment of crisis. The present might look depressing, but we must always remember that when the night is the darkest, sunlight will never be far behind.

Tomorrow was pregnant with possibilities, and the future lay ahead, waiting to be delivered. I said a silent prayer, crossed my fingers, and moved on to the next patient.

23
THE MEMORIES

"We saw you again,
We met you again.
In little Ayan.
'Dear Guri', you lived again
The way it was always meant to be,
The way you were destined to be,
But how we missed you ..."

Memories stir… they rise… they linger… and they smile.

Like brazen children, they test us with their impudence, sometimes painful, sometimes simply reminiscent.

But then, that's all they were – whimsical reminders of a memorable past, to be treated with patience, and sometimes pure indulgence.

And memories always hurt, just as they were doing today…

We had grown a year older, but he was frozen there, in time and in our memories.

Gurpreet would have turned thirty-eight today. His wife had called. Her son wanted to celebrate the day with his father's friends. We had to be with him.

Dr Gurpreet was a close friend and talked non-stop about the two 'loves' of his life – his paediatric ICU, and his four-year-old son. And whatever time he had left was spent ranting about his favourite dish – butter chicken!

Some people loved to eat. He lived to eat. A food fanatic, he never let even a morsel of food go waste. Much to the disgust of others, he could even pick it up from the floor and relish it. He always over-ordered, but would still enviously look at others' plates.

He belonged to a rural Punjabi family. When he cleared his medical entrance exams, his parents thought that their days of hardship were over. However, ten years down the line, he was still studying. First he did his MBBS, then completed an internship, then finished his MD, and finally did a fellowship in paediatric intensive care. His parents couldn't quite understand the medical jargon, but now after fifteen years that their son was finally earning money, they were happy and relieved, and looked forward to a comfortable life.

In between, Gurpreet had fallen in love, too, and married out of religion, much to their disapproval. However, he had a baby boy two years later, and things started settling down. He still cared a lot for the people from his native place. They kept visiting him whenever they were in trouble, especially when it concerned a medical emergency.

A year back, he had come with his cousin. She had been married for eight years but was still childless. He had brought her here for treatment. It was indeed a strange coincidence that though she had missed her periods many times earlier, this time when we checked, she turned out to be pregnant.

Her joy was a little restrained, and she chose not to believe it. I tried to reassure her, but ultimately, had to send her for an ultrasound. It confirmed that a new life was developing inside her. It took some time, but the happy news was finally sinking in. Gurpreet called me lucky for his sister. She was, naturally, apprehensive, and had a whole lot of queries.

It was almost lunchtime when I sent her home and decided to check with Dr Gurpreet. He was still busy with his patients. I was startled by a 'namaste', and turned to see Asha Devi sitting there with her one-year-old son Satyam. She was pointing us to him, and the hapless boy who could still not hold his neck, looked at me through his slanted eyes. He looked very beautiful, like most Down syndrome babies. His mother had triumphed against all odds to have him back from the hands of eternity.

Satyam had died three years back at the age of twenty, having drowned at Rishikesh. His mother was inconsolable. Already forty-five years of age, and her chances of future pregnancies permanently blocked with a sterilisation operation, her chances of having another baby looked dim. However, she was desperate. She wanted a recanalisation operation done to make her tubes patent once again. Considering her age, most doctors refused. However, her stubbornness saw her through. Satyam had to come back, so she got pregnant again – a testimony to her persistent efforts.

Dodging doctors who attempted to screen her for Down syndrome, she had landed up in our hospital just before the delivery. And baby Satyam, a reincarnate of the dead son, hardly fathoming the reason for his existence and unaware of the travails that awaited him, now grew, a little delayed, in the arms of the once-desolate parents. Destiny had been cruel, but this was Asha Devi's moment of reprieve. I couldn't help being a little critical still, I wished her well.

Gurpreet finished with his duties at the clinic and was more than happy to leave for lunch. The chicken and rice that I was carrying in my lunch box interested him as he sniffed hungrily. As always, he promised to get me the 'butter chicken' from his *pind* (village) in Punjab, and went on to tell me about some exotic recipes, such as chicken cooked in wine, that his wife had taught him. Like always, this was a bait in exchange for what lay inside somebody else's lunch box – a promise that would just tempt, but never be delivered. If life permitted, he would live and breathe chicken. His fast-expanding waistline had forced him to join a gym, but as always, he found a perfect excuse to stay away, in the garb of his profession. And oblivious to my angry looks, he became busy doing justice to a succulent piece of chicken. He ate as if there would be no tomorrow.

It was a relatively free day, and after winding up my work, I left early for home. These were moments to be treasured, the ones spent at home, for you never knew when you would be called back.

But Gurpreet had some other plans for me. His number flashed on my mobile. His cousin was puking badly. She had gone home, but every time she threw up, she rang him. And the poor guy, who was equally apprehensive, pinged me.

I assured him: 'It's all right. This is "nausea of pregnancy". It's actually a healthy sign. Relax!' He accepted that graciously, and passed on the message.

I was driving to my grocery shop when he rang for the fifth time. His repeated calls were now beginning to get on my nerves. Doctors were the worst patients! I did sound a little exasperated as I spoke to him, 'Guri, stop getting paranoid. She'll be fine. Let the pregnancy grow. Let's talk about this tomorrow!'

He immediately apologised, and I, too, was a little sorry for being easily ruffled.

There was a conference, two days later, that he was arranging. I teased him about wanting to have chicken biryani during lunch. He laughed. The menu was already fixed but he promised me biryani for the next conference. He thanked before calling off and didn't call again. I couldn't help feeling a tad bit relieved.

Gurpreet was on floor duty that day. The night went on at the usual pace. He remembered to speak to his wife and son, before they went to sleep. He made sure his wife read his son Ayan's favourite bedtime story, and promised Ayan his chocolates the next day. They had adjusted to his graveyard shifts, and his wife asked him to be home by eleven next day, as she had to be in the office by then. Ayan used to come back from the school a little later, and it was better if someone was home by then. He told her not to worry, but she always got jittery. He had a weird routine, but then inspite of being a non-medico, she was very supportive. And he loved her for all the sacrifices she had made by adjusting with him.

A small boy had been operated upon for a brain tumour about two days back, but things had turned complicated and he became brain-dead. The distraught parents wouldn't let go. He collapsed many times, but every time, he was somehow revived. Next morning, Gurpreet finished his rounds and, famished, went straight for breakfast with his friend, who like him specialised in intensive care. He was hungrily devouring some bread and cheese omelette, when his phone buzzed. The boy had suffered a cardiac arrest, again. This had become almost a routine every 9 am in the morning, but Gurpreet forgot everything at this call. He immediately left his breakfast and almost ran towards the ICU on the second floor. His friend followed him, repeatedly asking him to slow down. He avoided the lifts, rushing up the stairs as if something inside him was driving him towards the brain-dead child. Pushing open the heavy doors of the ICU, he reached the bedside of the little boy, and then to the horror of everyone present there, without saying a single word he just collapsed on the floor. His friend was almost breathless but right behind him. As if in a nightmare, he lifted Gurpreet up, found him pulseless and with no recordable blood pressure, deep into what is medically called 'shock'.

People collapsed in their homes, far away; were left on the roads seeking help; and took a long time to reach this very place. Some were saved and some declared 'reached late'. If one was destined to be saved, one couldn't have chosen a better place to collapse than here inside the ICU, with an intensivist behind, and put on a ventilator within minutes. Yet, this doctor who had saved many critically ill children, with a stubborn streak, lay helpless, suffering from a massive heart attack. His body played out the exact sequence of a 'shock'. The critical acid-base balance he was so fond of teaching, the blood gases that he bored us with details of, played havoc within him and taught him the final lessons.

He struggled on a ventilator with a grossly dilated heart, which had perhaps forgotten to contract. A ready cardiologist and a ready anaesthetist; the whole hospital fraternity crying for him; yet, our prayers could not revive him even once. His dear ICU equipment watched silently a failing young heart, as God denied them the privilege to save the one who had so confidently used and trusted them. A passionate intensivist, who thought arrogantly, that a good ventilator in a well-equipped ICU could never fail, lay in an irreversible hypoxic state. 'A heart was meant to beat, not rest!' he had once snorted, after struggling relentlessly and rising triumphant in reviving a child who had suffered a cardiac arrest. Oh, what a price he paid for his arrogance!

Somebody had to inform the unsuspecting wife, who was used to him not calling or reaching home on time. It is sad that we leave our homes for long hours of duty and forget to call our families, but they live with the trust that we are safe in our hospitals, believing that we are taking care of sick people there, but never imagining that we would ever fall critically sick ourselves. It would have never crossed her mind that he was unable to talk to her, not because he was busy, but because he was no more…

She was informed that he was not well and had to be admitted. It took a long time in the morning traffic rush, and by the time she reached, all efforts to revive him had failed. She was the wife of a doctor so she knew we must have tried our best, yet she was taken aback. The hospital had somehow failed her. We had no answers to the confusion that flooded her mind. A massive heart attack is what we explained to everyone else, but we were still reeling, at a loss to explain to ourselves, the 'whys' and the 'hows'.

His wife told us about his family history of recurrent early deaths of his maternal uncles, all suspected cases of heart attack.

He was an ardent foodie, with neither the time, nor the inclination to exercise. Being a doctor, he took things for granted. Maybe he trusted his hospital, or maybe he never thought that he could himself fall prey. He had been having chest pains off and on, but had ignored them. He had got an endoscopy done a week earlier, and the gastroenterologist had told him, specifically, that it was not acidity that plagued him. He needed to get his heart checked. However, the irresponsible patient neglected the doctor's advice. Few knew about this, except his wife, but she trusted him to take care of his health. His carelessness took away a promising doctor, a dear colleague and a friend, meeting an untimely end at a young age of thirty-seven.

Maybe he was unaware of the catastrophe that was brewing in his heart. The one always ready with answers, left the last questions unanswered.

Nevertheless, it exposed the perils of being overconfident, the price we pay for our unhealthy lifestyles, and the fact that the care providers also need to take care of their health. Above all, it taught us to cherish each moment of this unpredictable life. I could now fathom what patients like Asha Devi felt – the mad grief, the almost-physical pain, and the irreparable loss that makes you illogical.

His sister carried on with her pregnancy, not knowing her brother was no more. Her husband made her talk to me instead of Gurpreet, who, she had been told, was suddenly very busy these days. She felt it was odd, but by the time she got to know what had happened, she had been blessed with a son, who she and her husband named after him.

I was brought back to the present by the sound of Ayan's laughter, and I was surprised to see Gurpreet smiling at me. Life was never linear; it was circular. What was past, will be future, and what has gone, will come back one day. Ayan was a spitting image of his father, and, in him, my friend Guri lived again. I smiled back at him. Yes, life went on…

24
SOME UNRULY OBSESSIONS

"Some strange notions,
Some unruly obsessions,
And life turned,
A bundle of compulsions…"

There are times when you don't know whether to be irritated or to empathize. Meenu always put me in that spot. She would visit me with severe symptoms, which would be forgotten once she started speaking.

'Madam, you are like my elder sister. I was as educated as you. My father was very fond of teaching girls. However, Harpreet's family – you know – they didn't let me study further, and neither allowed me to work… made me sit at home.' She made a big face. 'Look at this bracelet. My father gave this to me. It is 30 gm, pure gold. He gives me so much jewellery. I was the richest *bahu* (daughter-in-law), from such a big family. However, my mother-in-law and her daughters hate me so much. They are always making me unhappy; never let me get close to my husband.'

She had a habit of flitting between topics. 'By the way, my husband wants me to go to Singapore with him. But I have refused!'

'Your mother-in-law, again?'

'Naah, my kids. How can I leave them?'

'They must be old enough now.' One was in college, another in high school.

'My son is home, these days. He has started looking so handsome, just like my brother. I have his pictures, and he sings well, too. He won a prize in a singing contest in his college. *Aapko dikhati hoon* (Let me show you).'

And she went on to show the pictures and videos of her kids, disregarding the patients waiting outside.

'You can leave them with your mother-in-law.'

Suddenly, she burst out crying. Ouch! Had I reminded her of some atrocity?

'My sister-in-law, Gurpreet's wife, is so smart. She has shifted to her own house. She never wanted to do any work at home. Yet, my mother-in-law doesn't speak badly of her. Neither does she go to stay with her.' Gurpreet was her husband's younger brother.

'Harpreet is so nice. He works hard, just to impress his mother. He has such a good business sense. He toils the whole day and brings money to the family, while others are just enjoying. Yet his mother, *uff* that lady! She creates so much trouble. She took away most of the things that my father gave me. Nobody in the family had ever brought a bigger dowry.' She lowered her voice suspiciously, and again I was told of that list of treasures she had brought. Patients waiting outside had started peeping in.

'Why do you people take so much dowry?' I felt compelled to ask.

'*Arre*, no ma'am. I don't believe in dowry at all. My brother just got married. We didn't ask for anything. *Na baba,* never! (Oh no, never!) Instead, we gave her so much jewellery and clothes. *Jo mere liye bana* (Whatever was made for me), my dad got that made for her, too. Yet, you know, how bad she is! She took all that and sent it to her mother. My poor brother! I don't know how he tolerates that woman.'

By now, I had understood that everyone was 'bad', except her and her side of the precious family. Almost half an hour had gone, but I still didn't know what her complains were.

'Meenu, can you tell me what brought you here today?' I could see the impatient faces waiting outside.

'Sorry, ma'am, you are like my elder sister. I need your blessings.'

Dramatically, she proceeded to touch my feet.

Older or younger, she always embarrassed me. It made me feel really awkward, blessing someone almost my age. However, I had no choice. She would have thrown a fit, had I not allowed her. This was now a routine. I had to listen to how vile her in-laws were, and how angelic her side of the family was. I had to repeatedly hear the list of treasures her father had sent. I still didn't understand if her husband was a demon, or if, outside his mother's influence, he became an angel. I had to listen to every detail about her children, see their pictures, and watch their videos. If I, at any point of time, did not, she would burst out crying. She kept her tears suspiciously close. Lately, I had started making excuses. Her husband also sympathised with me.

However, that was not how we had met. She used to always be in 'intractable pain', which was probably just an excuse to seek the attention of a husband who was either too busy, or fed up with her emotional outbursts.

One day, he let out his woes in front of me. She was hardly a wife to him, engrossed as she was in her children and parents. The rest of the time, her rants about his family came in between them. Things were bad, and often her husband got provoked to inflict physical violence. Domestic violence descended over their marriage like a pall of gloom and threatened to ruin her sanity. She needed some confidence-building, and he, some patience and restrain. Perhaps they both needed to cut their umbilical cords, and behave like a family, for the sake of their children.

I gained her trust when I chastised her husband for scolding and hitting such a sweet and innocent woman, who also happened to be the most educated one in the family. Fortunately, the repercussions of physical violence were not lost on him and they agreed to see a psychiatrist. Sessions of counselling helped, and they had, at least, reached a situation of peaceful co-existence. They had been married for seventeen years, but had still not been able to accept each other just as they were. However, it was indeed difficult growing out of the shadows they lived in. Meenu still mostly talked irrelevantly. At times, I didn't know who I pitied more.

But one thing was sure – she drained me mentally. I had my suspicions that she came just to talk to me. She hardly ever had any actual complains, but I still indulged her. Maybe she needed an outlet. In her own ways, she had become attached to this clinic, and it was difficult to push her out. Eventually, her husband had to come to my rescue every time.

My phone beeped. It was from the principal of a nearby school. Just yesterday, a group of teachers had brought in a small girl to the hospital. She was about eight years old. The teachers looked quite nervous. The girl had been found bleeding in the classroom by her teacher. That put them in a fix. The girl had not complained against anyone. There was no prima facie evidence of misconduct, either by anyone inside the school, or by anyone outside.

They had called up the parents immediately. The worried family rushed to the school, ready to blast the authorities. Her parents had already made up their mind to register a case against them, but the school also didn't want to take any chances. They took the child, along with her parents, to the nearest hospital. Soon, her relatives started pouring in. A preliminary examination showed no sign of any injury. The child looked neither mentally-disturbed, nor physically compromised. Rather, she kept behaving indifferently to the apprehensions of the adults staring at her. There were no telltale signs of sexual assault. No trace of bleeding could be seen, now. A child doesn't let you examine them well, and a detailed examination to rule out any internal injury was possible only under anaesthesia. However, the parents were not at all keen on that. Unfortunately, we couldn't give them any plausible reason for such a bleeding. They readily agreed to undergo an ultrasound examination. Given the circumstances, the manner in which the class teacher had handled the situation was highly commendable. The parents thawed a little and thanked the teacher for her efforts. They promised to report back if the bleeding recurred. The class teacher gave them a smile of gratitude and hugged the little girl, and they all left, relieved.

The principal couldn't thank us enough. It was tricky dealing with parents these days, but then it was equally tough for them, too. The apprehensions of the parents were also not totally unfounded as we live in an unpredictable world.

I, once again, complimented her school for giving quick medical aid to the child, and promptly rushing her to the hospital. They had not tried to downplay the incident, and had acted swiftly. Covering up an incident was tantamount to accepting guilt. Feeling happy, and promising to let me know about the girl's wellbeing, she put the phone down.

Appreciation is the best encouragement, and everyone loves being acknowledged.

Even I was no exception, I smiled to myself.

I finished the duties at my clinic fast. I had something waiting for me up in the labour room, and she was definitely not in a mood to either appreciate me, or indulge me.

'I have told you that I won't have a caesarean at any cost.'

She was in labour. With three previous pregnancy losses, and very little amniotic fluid inside, pointing towards a distressed baby, it was prudent to take her up for a caesarean section. Yet, she kept praying with the rosary beads in her hand, and refused for a surgical intervention. She was a patient, and it was not her prerogative to decide. There were things which were beyond either of our control. However, she had a guruji who had given her that chain of rosemary beads. He had assured her that everything would be all right this time, and she would deliver normally. She had been told that the doctors were mercenaries and whatever they did was guided by the greed for money. This was her brainwashed belief of us. Such patients spelt trouble, but then we were stuck with them.

Soon, she started having contractions and couldn't tolerate that, either. Neither pains, nor a caesarean section! It was good that we had the option of painless labour. Thankfully, she agreed and became more relaxed. A little later, the baby's heartbeat started dipping. Again, she was counselled to go for a surgery, but with her eyes fixed stubbornly on the rosary beads, she and her husband firmly declined. Fortunately, she progressed fast and was soon shifted into the labour room.

There, adding to our troubles, she decided to become totally hysterical. She would neither bear down, nor have a caesarean section. It was getting nightmarish. We were burning our bridges and yet, no voice of reason reached her. Left with only one option, we had no choice but to resort to assisted delivery, using forceps. The baby's heartbeat was dipping again. Some strained and stretched-out moments later, her baby was delivered. However, the stress that had started long back, had taken its toll. A compromised baby was born. It needed lot of resuscitation and was shifted to the neonatal ICU.

'All is well, doesn't always end well' in the medical field, especially obstetrics. And 'all that didn't end well' is, nevertheless, the doctor's fault. In today's age, both the internet-educated patients as well as the *baba*-guided ones, know better, but still, in the end, the blame is put squarely on the doctor. The baby was born hypoxic, critically brain-damaged as a consequence of prolonged stress, and at risk of suffering lifelong medical consequences. Even later, the parents remained in a state of denial. However, inspite of all this, the patient had our sympathies, and despite all our efforts, we suffered the blame.

If only there was some logic to the patient's obsession with the mode of delivery! From one, adamant for normal delivery, to another, going insane with fear and demanding a caesarean, the line between the clinician and the patient had started to blur. Maybe we needed to respect the boundaries a little more, and in all humility, we doctors needed to try harder to understand their hostile mentalities.

At times, our professional fee becomes the bone of contention, but then what choice does one have in a private practice? Even a guruji took a decent amount of *dakshina* (payment) these days, but they still had their unshakeable trust.

A new life suffered disastrously, while the adults simply tried to shrug off their accountability. Wisdom doesn't come easily to those with misplaced loyalties and trust. Too much loyalty stemmed from fear, and made one dependent. Hopefully, one day they would introspect and understand.

A small blood vessel closed in the heart, and a hair grew grey, silently. Obstetrics was unpredictable and stressful. I needed to wash it all away with a hot cup of tea. And then it was time to call it a day...

ABOUT THE AUTHOR

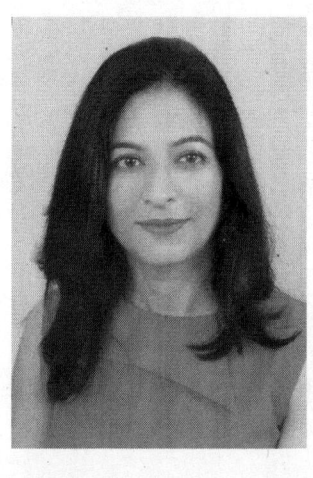

Tripti Sharan is a gynaecologist and obstetrician by profession, and a writer by choice. She works as a senior consultant at BLK Super Speciality Hospital in New Delhi, India.

Writing is her passion and refuge. She recently published her book of poetry, *The Dewdrops ... a journey begins*, which was adjudged the best anthology in English poetry (2015) by 'Aagman' literary group. She has also contributed short stories and poems to many anthologies. She is currently working on her next book, *The anecdotes of a medico*, an interesting take on the life of a medical student, as well as another volume of her poems.

An ardent swimmer and a fitness freak, she learned the value of healthy eating and physical exercise when she lost her mother to a lifestyle disease four years ago. Observing and interacting with people is one of her favourite pastimes

Health, gender and socio-political concerns are issues close to her heart. She is actively involved in social work and in promoting creativity among the masses. Reaching out to people and inspiring them through her writings is her way of giving back something to the beautiful world that she lives in. She's married to a paediatric intensivist, and is a mother to two adolescent boys. Pursuing her passion and profession together is akin to constantly living on the edge, but it only serves to inspire her to write more and share more. When she is neither writing nor practicing in the hospital, she loves to listen to music, read books, or spend time idling with her family.

According to her, she doesn't see 'patients' in her clinic, she sees 'emotions'. Behind every emotion breathes a story, and every story deserves to be told.

As a doctor she gets to see them at their most vulnerable times, and these moments are both inspirational and revealing. It is her utmost desire to share with people the myriad issues that plague women in India.

Though it is 'motherhood' that draws a woman to her clinic, it is 'womanhood' that inspires her to write. In a country where a 'mother' has always been celebrated, she seeks out the 'woman' who suffers in anonymity. For ages, the mother-son relationship has been revered, and daughters ignored. No wonder the present is scarred by the wounds of the past.

As she tries to pen the different hues of women, a question boldly stares at her – is a woman's sexuality indeed her nemesis? It rises to taunt again and again. She searches for the answer in every story, but fails. She leaves it to the readers to make their own interpretation.

Maybe the reader can identify with someone in this book, or the characters may sound familiar. For in here, one meets the most sacrificing and most loving of species that God has ever made. They are called women! Yet, for the majority of those who suffer from complexities beyond comprehension, this book is just a feeble attempt to touch their lives.